Fire Over Heathrow

By the same author

Dambuster A Life of Guy Gibson VC – 1994
She Who Dared (with Jackie George) – 1999
Violette Szabo the Life that I Have – 2002
Hitler's Traitors – 2003
Fly With The Stars (co-author Ian Ottaway) – 2007

Fire Over Heathrow

The Tragedy of Flight 712

Susan Ottaway

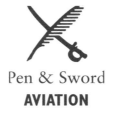

Pen & Sword
AVIATION

First published in Great Britain in 2008 by
Pen & Sword Aviation
an imprint of
Pen & Sword Books Ltd
47 Church Street
Barnsley
South Yorkshire
S70 2AS

Typeset in Palatino Linotype by
Lamorna Publishing Services.

Printed and bound in England by Biddles Ltd.

Pen & Sword Books Ltd. incorporates the imprints of Pen & Sword
Aviation, Pen & Sword Maritime, Pen & Sword Military, Wharncliffe
Local History, Pen & Sword Select, Pen & Sword Military Classics
and Leo Cooper.

For a complete list of Pen & Sword titles please contact
PEN & SWORD BOOKS LIMITED
47 Church Street, Barnsley, South Yorkshire, S70 2AS, England
E-mail: enquiries@pen-and-sword.co.uk
Website: www.pen-and-sword.co.uk

For Ian

Contents

My desk in Windsor Castle looks eastwards towards London Airport. In the beautifully clear late afternoon of 8 April 1968, I noticed a Boeing 707 flying south, straight and level, between the Castle and Heathrow. It struck me as odd, since most flights taking-off to the west climb quite steeply as they turn to the south, or they come fairly close past the Castle going west. I also noticed, what I first thought, was the sun being reflected from the side of the aircraft. It then dawned on me that it was not the reflection of the sun, but that one of the engines was on fire.

I followed the aircraft with binoculars as it turned over Slough, where the burning engine fell off, and then until it disappeared from view as it landed on Runway 05. I lost sight of the aircraft, but almost immediately a cloud of black smoke appeared, and I could not help wondering whether the passengers and crew had been able to escape.

This book is about that fateful flight, and about what happened after it landed. This is an account of that crash, and of the remarkable heroism of Barbara Jane Harrison, for which she was posthumously awarded the George Cross. It is a tragic, but also an inspiring story.

Acknowledgements

When, during the Blitz, King George VI wanted to honour ordinary men and women who had displayed great bravery, he felt that there was no suitable award that he could give. He wanted something that would be equivalent to the ultimate military decoration and so instituted a new medal, the George Cross, which came into being by Royal Warrant on 24 September 1940. It was, and remains to this day, the highest civilian award; equal in status to the Victoria Cross.

Some time ago, while doing research for a biography of Violette Szabo, I discovered that, although several recipients of other medals have had their awards replaced by the George Cross, there have only ever been four directly granted to women. Of these, three were given to Special Operations Executive agents in France during the Second World War. Odette Sansom received her medal herself; the other two were awarded posthumously to Noor Inayat Khan and Violette Szabo after they had been executed in Nazi concentration camps – the former in Dachau and the latter in Ravensbrück. The fourth, and only peacetime award of the George Cross to a woman, was to a pretty, fun-loving stewardess who worked for the state-owned airline, BOAC. Her name was Barbara Jane Harrison and she was just six weeks short of her twenty-third birthday when the accident, for which she was honoured, took place.

Noor Inayat Khan, Odette Sansom and Violette Szabo, have all had books written about them. Although Jane, as she was known to family and friends, has been mentioned in articles about the accident in 1968, and in books about the George Cross, she has not been remembered with a book about the incident and the part that she played, and very little is known about her at all.

The year 2008 marks the fortieth anniversary of the tragedy in which Jane Harrison lost her life trying to save the lives of others. A book about her and about what happened is long overdue.

When I appealed for information from eyewitnesses to the accident and from surviving passengers, I received a letter from Keith Payne who, as a small boy, had watched from his garden as the pilot made his desperate attempt to get the jet airliner back to Heathrow before it exploded and killed everyone on board. The account of what he saw appears later in the book but a comment he made about the award of the George Cross to Jane Harrison struck me as being exactly right and I felt that I had to include it. He said:

> A couple of years ago I read the citation for Barbara Harrison's George Cross. I suppose it will never be known if she succumbed whilst trying to extricate that disabled passenger or returned to be with him [*sic*] until the fire fighters arrived. ... Whilst I would not wish to take anything away from the three other women awarded the George Cross, this was different. They were in occupied France fighting an enemy in a time when the ultimate sacrifice must have always been in the mind. This was peacetime and a day that was perfectly normal until it all went awfully wrong. Under those circumstances, such courage is exceptional.

It is impossible to disagree with Mr Payne's opinion. This was an ordinary day for the young stewardess. She got up that morning with no thought for the danger that she would face later in the day. Unlike the three SOE women there *was* no danger to be expected, just a day at work, even though her work was unusual, taking her, as it did, to exotic places around the world. At the end of that day she anticipated being able to spend some pleasant free time with the rest of the crew before the next leg of their flight to Australia. She had everything to look forward to and nothing to fear and yet, later that afternoon, she died in the blazing wreck of the aircraft in which she was working. She could easily have escaped but instead chose to try and save the lives of the four passengers who were still on board.

She was a remarkable young woman. There are many people who are still alive today because of what Labour politician, Anthony Crosland, called 'her lonely and courageous action'.

The story of Jane Harrison and the tragic accident that killed her, should not be forgotten.

When embarking on a project such as this an author has to rely heavily on the assistance of the family and friends of the people concerned as well as eyewitnesses, work colleagues, museums and archives.

Although the events described happened in the 1960s and the people concerned live all over the world, the response to my requests for help has been enormous and the men and women who have contacted me have done so with tremendous enthusiasm. Many shared my belief that Jane Harrison's story should be told but, as I listened to their accounts of what had happened all those years ago, I realized that Jane's story would not be complete without including those of the people with whom she had shared those few moments of horror on that sunny April afternoon. Many of their tales were heartbreaking; I know what it must have cost them to share them with me. Many times as I read about, or listened to what they had been through I found myself in tears. They, too, are remarkable people.

***

My first expression of appreciation must go to HRH The Duke of Edinburgh. I am truly honoured that His Royal Highness consented to write the foreword to this book and thank him most sincerely.

***

It was not possible to find everyone that I sought. I contacted the fire service and the police and received charming letters in reply to my request for information. Sadly, in both cases, that information was no longer available and none of the people who had worked in those services in 1968 was still in their employment. Staff at the two hospitals who looked after the passengers from Whisky Echo, were very helpful but, again, could find no one still working there who had been involved in the care of the survivors.

Strangely, several letters and e-mails to various departments of British Airways, which was formed in 1974 by the merger of BEA and BOAC, were not even acknowledged, including one sent to the press office, at an address given on the airline's website as being specifically for journalists with media enquiries.

Although I managed to contact more crew members from Whisky Echo than I thought would be possible, I wasn't able to find them all. All, except one, of those that I did find gave me a wonderful insight into what it was like on Flight 712. The one exception did not want to have to relive the events of forty years ago and I understand this completely. The stories of those I didn't manage to contact have been taken from recollections of the other crew members, records of interviews given at the time and official reports held at the National Archives.

I am so grateful to everyone who has contributed with information, photos, contact details, eyewitness accounts of the accident to Flight 712 and numerous other kindnesses. For the special part you have each played in making this book possible I would like to thank: Ian Anderson, Richard Argyle, John Avery, G. Barber, Damian Baston, Alan Bishop, Allan Blackman, Gillie Blake, Vic Buck, Peter Campbell, Ric Chaplin, Lesley Cosgrove, Richard Daniels, Ann Davidson, John Davidson, Hubert Day, Nickie Dean, Kevin Dent, Savio d'Souza, Sue Dutton, Jim Edwards, Sheila Ferguson, Captain E.D. 'Wyn' Fieldson, Reg Findlay, Janice Fitzpatrick, Audrey Ford, Jez Gale, Ken Gibson, Jennifer Gill, Peter Groves, Richard Haigh, Keith Harris, Malcolm Harvey, Pat Heselden, Brigadier Sir Miles Hunt-Davis, Robin Johnson, Tricia Jolly, Mandeep Juttla, Ewan Larcombe, Audrey M. Lendon, Katherin Looke, David

Macdougald, Amanda Mizza, Kjell Nilsson, Sheila O'Sullivan, Sue Palmer, Keith Payne, Walter Phillips, Josephine Pole, Lindsay Puddifoot, Hazel Randall, Tim Rayner, Glynn Rogers, Gary Simpson, Colin Smith, Vic Smith, Phil Southcott, Brian Stainer, Roy Stannett, Bob Steed, Arthur Thorning, John 'Tom' Toy, Dacre Watson, Val Weir, John Wegg, Dave Welch, Mick West, Stan Wilkinson and Katherine Williamson.

Thanks also to the editors of the newspapers in the UK and Australia who kindly printed my requests for help.

Barry Ballard, Doug Cotterell, Jim Davies, Keith Hayward and Gill Sparrow, at the British Airways Museum, volunteer their valuable time to run the museum and their expertise and knowledge have, once again, proved invaluable.

Doctors Roger Green and Roy Maclaren very kindly gave me information about their work in aviation medicine and the Barbara Harrison Prize, and Professor Helen Muir allowed me to quote from her work on passenger safety in transport aircraft; I am very grateful to them all.

Pete Bish and Celia Kunert put me in touch with both Frank Tyler, who very kindly allowed me to use his dramatic photo on the cover, and John Davis, the air traffic controller who looked after Whisky Echo from the ground during the short time it was airborne. I am grateful to Pete and Celia as I am to Frank and John. Thanks also to John's wife Jaqi for persuading her husband to allow me to use the photo of him with his MBE at Buckingham Palace.

Mrs Diddy Davis-Gordon and Mrs Audrey Taylor very kindly shared their memories of their late husbands, Chief Steward Neville Davis-Gordon and Captain Cliff Taylor. As Mrs Davis-Gordon said, 'It's what my husband would have wanted'.

I have been extremely fortunate to have been able to speak to, and correspond with, several crew members from Flight 712. Special thanks are due to Stewardess Rosalind Chatterley née Unwin and her husband, Nick; Steward Andrew McCarthy and his wife, Christina; First Officer Francis Kirkland, and Acting First Officer John Hutchinson and his wife, Sue. John not only shared his memories of Whisky Echo with me, he also offered, in his role as Past Master of the Guild of Air Pilots and Air

Navigators, to contact HRH The Duke of Edinburgh to ask him if he would consider writing the foreword to the book and for this, too, I am very grateful.

Although I hoped to contact some of the passengers from Flight 712 I was not confident of finding any after so many years. Several, however, have been most considerate in sharing their memories with me and lending me photos. They are Eric Blower, Brian and Shirley Cooper, Dr Richard Hamond, who took the photo which appears on the back of the book, Trevor Hay, Fred and Vera Pragnell and Mark Wynter. Basil Henn also kindly told me about his father, Canon Wilfrid Henn and his mother Georgina, who were also passengers on the flight. I know that it has been difficult for some of them to relive their experiences and I thank them all for their generosity in doing so.

Jane Harrison's friends and family have also been generous in sharing with me their memories and anecdotes of the brave girl who meant so much to them. Even after all this time they have spoken about her with great enthusiasm and affection, reliving those days when she was a part of their day-to-day lives, as if it were only yesterday. Her friends are Dawn Bailey, Kay Haw née Golightly, Margaret Jessop, Michael Moore, Sheila Walkington née Turton and her cousin is Patrick Worthington. Very special thanks to Sue Buck, Jane Harrison's sister, for her patience in answering my questions, for suggesting areas of research, for copying letters written to her family after Jane's death, for putting me in touch with Jane's friends, for supplying photos and for the many, many more kindnesses that she has shown to me. I know that it has been difficult for her at times too but I hope that she will think it has been worthwhile in the end.

My final thanks are to my partner, Nick, for his constant support and help, and to my brother, Ian, for the beautifully drawn map, illustrating Whisky Echo's position during its short flight, and for all his help with the project. I couldn't have done it without you both!

Susan Ottaway

2008

Glossary

ACJMS – Air Corporations Joint Medical Service – the air corporations being BOAC and BEA.
ATCO – Air Traffic Control Officer
BAA – British Airport Authority
BEA – British European Airways
BOAC – British Overseas Airways Corporation
BOT – Board of Trade
EO – Engineer Officer
FO – First Officer
GMC – Ground Movement Controller
HOLDING POINT – The place where the aircraft waits for clearance from air traffic control to take-off.
IAL – International Aeradio Ltd
ILS – Instrument Landing System
LAS – London Ambulance Service
LATCC – London Air Traffic Control Centre
LFB – London Fire Brigade
LINE UP – To position the aircraft at the end of the runway with its nose wheel on the runway's centre line, ready for take-off.
MAYDAY – An international radiotelephone signal word used by aircraft and ships in distress. (From the French m'aider – help me!)
Mc – Megacycle
MT – Motor Transport
PAR – Precision Approach Radar
Qantas – Queensland and Northern Territory Air Service – the Australian national airline.

RCP – Royal College of Physicians

rendezvous point – designated areas where emergency service vehicles were sent to await the arrival of aircraft making unscheduled landings at Heathrow due to onboard emergencies.

R/T – Radio telephony

RVR – Runway Visual Range

THRESHOLD – The start of the usable part of a runway for landing. This is marked by a single white line on visual runways and by eight longitudinal parallel white lines, four each side of the runway centreline on runways with ILS facilities.

THRUST REVERSER – a device to reverse the thrust of a jet engine to enable braking on an aircraft.

TWA – Trans World Airways

USAF – United States Air Force

VHF – Very High Frequency

Introduction

The event about which this book is written happened forty years ago, in April 1968. The penultimate year of the Swinging Sixties, 1968 was a year of violence and change, described by acclaimed American journalist, Mark Kurlansky, as 'The Year that Rocked the World'.[1]

The Vietnam war was still raging and the year began with the Tet offensive in which the North Vietnamese communist forces attacked cities in the south of the country. American and South Vietnamese troops retaliated the following month with a murderous bloodbath that wiped out many of their enemies and shocked the world in its ferocity. In March Lyndon B. Johnson announced he would not stand for re-election as President of the United States in November and, when the elections took place, Republican Richard M. Nixon beat Democrat Hubert H. Humphrey to become the thirty-seventh president of the United States and one of the most controversial of modern times.

At the end of March the world's first spaceman, Soviet cosmonaut Yuri Gagarin, died in an air crash and, on 4 April, in the city of Memphis, Tennessee, civil rights leader, Dr Martin Luther King, was assassinated.

In mid April students in Germany rioted, following the shooting and wounding of left-wing student leader Rudi Dutschke. The riots soon spread and, in May, French students participated in even bigger riots and were soon joined by French workers who staged strikes forcing President Charles de Gaulle to announce a referendum and a programme of reforms.

Robert F. Kennedy, the brother of assassinated US President

John F. Kennedy was, himself, assassinated in June by a Jordanian immigrant, Sirhan B. Sirhan.

Following Czech Communist leader Alexander Dubcek's liberal reforms, Soviet troops had been massing on the country's border and, in August, invaded Czechoslovakia, crushing Dubcek's government and imposing severe restrictions that reversed the democratic reforms. Czech citizens demonstrated against the invasion and, across Europe, protest marches took place but to no avail. When the tanks left the country in September, Czechoslovakia was, once more, under the Soviet thumb.

The atmosphere of gloom should have been lifted when the Games of the XIX Olympiad were held in Mexico City in October but that event too was cloaked in controversy; first because of the killing of hundreds of student rioters just before the opening of the games and then by the Black Power clenched-fist salutes of some of the black American athletes.

In a Britain beset with economic problems, the ruling Labour party began to lose parliamentary seats in by-elections, the Foreign Secretary George Brown resigned, as a protest against what he considered to be Prime Minister Harold Wilson's dicta-torial style and, in the House of Commons, a bill restricting Asian immigration was introduced.

On 7 April British motor racing enthusiasts were saddened to learn of the death of Formula One racing driver Jim Clark in Hockenheim, West Germany. Then, in the late afternoon of the following day, came news of an air accident which wiped all other news off the front pages of the nation's newspapers.

**

In the Thameside village of Wraysbury, close to Heathrow airport, Val Weir was taking her twin daughters out in their pram. As she walked along the road Val, an ex BOAC stew-ardess, heard the sound of an aircraft and casually glanced up to see what it was. Something about the sound was wrong and she was horrified to see flames coming from one of the engines on the port wing of a BOAC Boeing 707. Finding herself outside the house of an ex BEA stewardess that she knew, she called out to her friend and the two women watched as the flames on the wing steadily got worse and they saw the engine fall off the wing. Val remembers yelling 'The pod's fallen off, the pod's fallen off...' Fearing that it had fallen into the middle of the nearby town of Staines, they telephoned the fire brigade to alert them to the situation and were taken aback when, a few minutes later, a fire engine came round the corner into the road, looking for the fire. After a quick explanation, the fire crew turned their engine around and rushed off towards Heathrow.

Val and her friend stood watching the burning aircraft as it turned back towards Heathrow airport and until it disappeared from view. Moments later, a pall of thick, black smoke rose high into the sky.

Chapter 1

Early Days

Alan Harrison was the youngest of four children, and the only boy. He had been educated at Woodhouse Grove Public School in Leeds. After his mother died, his father remarried and moved to Placeville, California, where he made his money by buying and selling stocks and shares. He, however, along with many others, lost his money in the Wall Street crash of October 1929. Times were hard and money was short but, with so many people in reduced circumstances, work was not easy to find.

Alan's step-mother, Dorothy, became a nanny and was fortunate to eventually find a position with the family of Charlie Chaplin, looking after his children. Her husband was also offered a job by the film star and went to work for him as his gardener.

Before finding a permanent job and settling down himself, Alan made a trip to America to visit his father and step-mother and their daughter who was born in America and was named Angela. It was an exciting time for the good-looking young man, who bore more than a passing resemblance to Hollywood actor, Errol Flynn. He travelled around and experienced a life that most people only dream of and his visit stretched from weeks to months and then to years.

After he had been in America for six years he began to miss his homeland and decided that he did not want to remain in America for the rest of his life. He returned to England and settled back in Yorkshire, becoming a constable with the Bradford City Police.

Soon after his return he met a pretty girl called Lena Adlard at a dancing class and soon the couple started to go out together.

The relationship blossomed, they became engaged and were married in 1936. Five years later they became parents for the first time when their daughter, Susan Elizabeth – Sue – was born.

By May 1945 Lena and Alan Harrison had every reason to be happy. They had survived the war, they had a lovely daughter, by then four years old, and Lena was about to give birth to their second child who was expected later that month.

Two weeks after VE Day, on 24 May, Barbara Jane Harrison was born at the family home in Kingsdale Crescent, Bradford, Yorkshire. Although her parents named her Barbara she was always known to family and friends as Jane.

Despite being English by birth, Lena was of Italian descent. Her grandmother, Josephina, was Italian born but had come to live in England at the age of three and, when she grew up and married, she chose a fellow Italian.

Lena had worked for furriers Swears and Wells before having her children but she was not in good health. She suffered from rheumatoid arthritis which sometimes left her so incapacitated that she was unable to do anything at all. The drugs she was given for her illness brought their own problems and the young mother found life with two small children very difficult. She had to rely on her own mother for help and it was she who did a lot of the housework in the Harrison household when the girls were small.

When it was time for Sue to go to school Alan and Lena enrolled her at a private school called Greystones, in Bradford; four years later Jane joined her there. Both girls were brought up as Roman Catholics, their mother's religion and, after she left Greystones, Sue went to St Josephs' College. Jane stayed at Greystones until, believing that the sea air might help his sick wife, Alan Harrison moved the family to Scarborough. Jane was enrolled at Newby County Primary School on the north-west outskirts of Scarborough, close to the family's new home and Sue went to the Convent of Ladies of Mary in Scarborough.

Despite their mother's illness the girls had a happy life with lots of playmates and family to visit. Their father's eldest sister, Jean, and her husband Giles Worthington, who lived in

Ormskirk, had three sons, Patrick, Alan and Martin. The girls also had cousins Robin, Carol and Richard, the children of their Aunt Kit. They sometimes spent days out together and the family photo albums record happy times in places such as Southport, and holidays in Wales.

By the summer holidays of 1955 Lena had become very ill and the girls were sent to stay with Aunt Jean and her family. When the holidays came to an end and they returned to Scarborough they found that, during their absence, their mother had died. The drugs she had been prescribed to treat her rheumatoid arthritis had affected her kidneys causing nephritis which had made her legs swell and eventually contributed to her death at the age of forty-one. There can be nothing harder for a child to cope with than the loss of a parent so early in life. Sue was only fourteen and Jane just ten years old when Lena died and they had not even had the chance to say goodbye to her or to attend her funeral. Life would never be the same for them again.

Alan Harrison was a good father and his daughters were very fond of him but it was difficult for him to work and bring up two girls by himself. He tried to keep their routines as normal as possible but, inevitably, the girls, especially Sue, had to grow up much faster than most of their friends. When the others were outside playing or visiting each other, Sue and Jane had their household chores to do. Most of the burden of keeping the house running while their father was at work fell to Sue, as Jane had a knack of disappearing whenever it was time for her to do something that she didn't like. To minimize the amount of time that the girls – mainly Sue – had to spend in the kitchen at weekends, their father decided that they would have their traditional Sunday lunch on a Saturday and then on Sunday have the leftovers so that they had at least one day free from the need to cook.

When Jane passed her 11 Plus exam she went to Scarborough Girls High School where she met the girls who would be her friends for the rest of her short life. Sheila Turton, one of those girls, recalled that when the new term started Jane was missing. She was not sure why she had not started on the same day as everyone else but said:

The teachers called her name so often she was almost a celebrity when she finally appeared. How do girls who have nothing in common but passing the eleven plus, sort themselves out so quickly after the initial shakedown? Jane was fun. She never seemed daunted by anyone. Jane made fun of everything and everybody. Nothing was sacred. We were labelled 'naughty' but compared to girls today we were paragons of virtue.

When the nuns at the Convent of Ladies of Mary heard that Sue Harrison's younger sister was now attending a secular school they were horrified and told Sue that she must tell her father to move Jane to the convent immediately. Sue was not at all comfortable with the task she had been set, feeling that it was not her place to instruct her father but did tell him what the nuns had said. Jane remained at Scarborough Girls High!

Margaret Jessop also began her secondary education at the same time as Jane and the girls became firm friends. Margaret had just lost her father and so she and Jane had something in common. As Margaret says:

> With hindsight I realise how much 'easier' it is to lose a father than a mother, if you can call it easy, as I remember Jane at 11 having to take the washing to the launderette, do the shopping and generally grow up; things which I never had to do. I also remember her father once burning all her makeup for some reason; I'm sure he was worried out of his mind with the responsibility.
>
> However despite all this, she was so much fun to be with, always had new ideas of things to do and games to play.

Kay Golightly, along with Sheila, Margaret and Jane formed a little gang. Her memories of those schooldays were that they were always together and often in trouble with their headmistress, Miss Woods. Their misdemeanours were fairly innocuous but, at a time when running in the corridors or talking while going up or down the stairs was frowned upon, the gang was considered to be rather wild and its members were frequently castigated in front of the entire school during the morning assembly.

Kay remembers one incident where Miss Woods announced:

Never before in the history of the school have the police been called to investigate two girls stealing. Kay Golightly and Jane Harrison report to me.

The crime that the police were investigating was the stealing of some ripe cherries which the pair had picked from trees along the side of the road. Their partners in crime were council gardeners who were working nearby and who helped the girls fill their berets with the fruit. Oblivious to the fact that the entire episode had been witnessed by their geography teacher, they climbed aboard the bus to go home and began munching on the cherries. The next morning came the public shaming during assembly. Luckily for Jane her father was no longer a policeman so he had not been embarrassed at work by his younger daughter's behaviour.

This situation did not last however as, after leaving the police force, Alan Harrison had become a driving examiner. One evening when the girls were supposed to be revising for their GCE 'O' levels, Kay decided to borrow her mother's moped and take Jane for a ride along the Scarborough seafront. All went well until the pair were stopped by a policeman outside the Futurist Theatre in Foreshore Road. The constable wanted to see Kay's licence and proof of insurance which he, of course, knew she did not have. The girls were given a good dressing down by him, witnessed by the 'Black and White Minstrels' who were taking a break between shows on the roof of the theatre, and were made to walk home pushing the moped – a distance of about three miles. The constable threatened to inform their headmistress and said that Kay would be fined, not only for having no licence or insurance but also for taking Jane as a passenger. Kay's parents and Jane's father were informed and the girls were grounded. It didn't improve Alan Harrison's reputation as a driving examiner to have his underage daughter, and her equally underage friend, flitting around Scarborough on a moped but it didn't harm his career either as, when he eventually retired, it was from a senior position in the Department of Transport.

Kay remembers Jane's father as being a shy but extremely nice man. He once took the girls' form teacher out for tea but made the huge mistake of taking Jane and her friends along as well. The outing was not a success with the girls giggling and prodding each other under the table, and it was not something that he chose to repeat.

Sheila also remembered Alan Harrison dating the teacher:

> He was a handsome man, I realise now, and often had a girl friend (much to Jane's amusement/embarrassment) and even dated one of our teachers which Jane thought a huge joke. She was a lovely teacher and we all loved her. I think her name was Miss Verity and she taught History.
>
> I remember Jane telling us about a visit to the Floral Hall which was a theatre hosting the old summer variety shows which, in the 50s, attracted huge stars. Some performers needed audience participation and Jane was embarrassed because her dad insisted in clapping along and shouting out. Of course the retelling was probably much funnier than the actual event.

Despite her high spirits which were often judged to have been misdirected, Jane's schooldays weren't entirely marred by getting into scrapes. Although she could not be described as a robust child she enjoyed sport and played rounders, hockey and netball at Scarborough Girls High School. She and Kay also played cricket for the local village ladies team as they lived close to each other, while Sheila and Margaret both lived on the same street in town. While at her primary school Jane had been a Brownie and was later a Girl Guide which, Kay believes, instilled in her, 'a strong sense of duty and a caring nature'.

When Sue Harrison was seventeen she left the convent and went to study agriculture at Bishop Burton college. Jane was thirteen at the time so, with her sister away at college and having no mother to help ease her through her teenage years, she spent a lot of time at the homes of her friends. She was often at the Golightly house where she was welcomed by Kay's mother and was regarded by Kay, herself, as a sister. Sheila's parents had a 'soft spot' for her too and her mother once made a dress for Jane when she was making one for Sheila which was a 'big event' as, according to Sheila, she 'was not the most maternal of creatures'.

Kay's mother enjoyed dressmaking and made a lot of full skirts with net petticoats for Kay and for Jane too. The girls learnt to dance at the local Dance Rooms, going primarily to get to know the boys who also attended and, although the dancing was mainly ballroom, the last session was jiving which they both enjoyed and which allowed them to show off their stylish outfits. They practised jiving at Jane's house with their school uniform ties, looped round door handles, used as 'partners'. Jane had a blue Dansette record player – a highly prized item in the 1950s and 60s – and they danced while playing her favourite records on it. Over forty years later Kay has strong memories of that time whenever she hears those favourites: Elvis Presley's *Jailhouse Rock*, Cliff Richard singing *Move It* or *Summer Holiday*, Bobby Vee's *Take Good Care of my Baby*, the Everly Brothers' *Cathy's Clown* and *Be Bop A Lula* , Buddy Holly's *It Doesn't Matter Anymore* and *It's Only Make Believe* by Conway Twitty.

The girls also listened to music from a jukebox while doing their homework in a local coffee bar, their books spread out next to cups of frothy coffee on the yellow Formica table tops. Even this seemingly innocent pastime was viewed with disapproval by the staff at Scarborough Girls High.

A more serious infringement of school discipline occurred when the 'gang' decided to colour their hair with the latest products obtained from the chemists shop owned by Margaret's mother. Using such colours as African Violet and Chestnut Sheen, all four girls went to school one morning each sporting a different hair colour. Jane had chosen green! This bit of harmless fun earned them all order marks and, no doubt, odd looks from passers-by.

Jane's school friends and her sister, Sue, all recalled her love of animals. While living in Scarborough she kept cats, guinea pigs and hens. Sue's friend Anne remembered that Jane was once in trouble with her father when she let her cats run around on the kitchen worktops. But despite their odd differences Jane and her father were close. He seems to have shared her liking for animals as one day when they were in Filey they found the owner of the ponies who gave rides on the beach during the summer and asked him what happened to them when the holiday season was over. Finding that they were put out to grass, they decided to bring two of them home and put them out to graze for the winter in a nearby field. Although done with the best of intentions they had to return them soon afterwards when the hungry horses had eaten every scrap of grass in the field. Sue remembered, too, the black and white family cat, and the white mice that Jane had secretly obtained and kept in a cage under her bed.

For most of her life Jane took photos which she put into her own photo album, each one carefully captioned. An outgoing, friendly girl she spent a lot of her holidays as a teenager on trips to Europe which were arranged through the World Friends group. The young people visited countries such as Holland, Germany and Austria and, by the time she left school, Jane was very well-travelled, more so than most of her contemporaries in those days. Sue recalled one trip that Jane made – she believes it was to Vienna – when instead of having a lot of fun with her friends, she was separated from them and only met up with them again a few days before returning to England. The photo album recorded many of these trips with images of the places she visited and the people she met.

In 1961 just before Jane was due to sit her 'O' level GCEs her father was transferred to Doncaster. Jane stayed on in Scarborough until her exams were over and then joined him in Doncaster where, in September, she enrolled at Doncaster High School. She again began to fill the house with animals and on a trip to Doncaster market one day bought two cats from the pet stall. They cost 7/6 and 5/- respectively and Jane named them Geoffrey Douglas and Agnes. She managed to keep them in her bedroom for three weeks before her father discovered that he had lodgers but they eventually became family fixtures, remaining with Alan Harrison after Jane had left home and only being given new homes when Alan, himself, moved down south to live in Pinner in Middlesex. Several black and white photos of Geoffrey Douglas and Agnes remain in Jane's photo album to this day.

By the Easter holidays of 1962 Jane had not yet decided whether she should stay on at school or get a job. She attended an interview for a job at Martin's Bank (now the Yorkshire Bank) in the town and when it was offered to her decided to take it. A few days after starting work she wrote a letter to her headmistress explaining that she wouldn't be coming back to school and telling her that her new job was very hard work but that she liked it. Kay remembers that at the end of each working day Jane had to balance her books and was often late leaving for home as she frequently had to rework all her figures before getting them to balance.

At around this time her three friends also started work; Margaret went to the Halifax Building Society while Sheila and Kay became civil servants. In the back of her mind Kay regarded her job as temporary as she had decided that she wanted to become an air hostess.

Sheila had moved to Leeds where she shared a flat with her sister. She and Jane became very close at this time and Jane sometimes spent weekends at the flat where she met John, Sheila's boyfriend and later husband, and their crowd of friends. As Sheila says:

It was the Swinging Sixties and, boy, did we swing!

Chapter 2

The Birth of Whisky Echo

At the beginning of 1962 a Boeing 707-420 rolled off the production line at the company's west coast plant at Seattle, Washington. The aircraft was given the designation 707-465; 707-4 to demonstrate that it was a 707-420 series and 65 to show which company had ordered it. The number 65 was the customer identification allocated by Boeing to the British company, Cunard-Eagle.

Cunard-Eagle had applied for, and been given, a licence to operate a service between London and New York in direct competition with the state-owned airline, BOAC, and had ordered two Boeing 707s to use on the new route. It had been a landmark decision by the licensing board as an independent airline had never before been granted a licence for a route already operated by a state-run company. BOAC was not pleased with the board's decision. Cunard-Eagle would be taking away some of its passengers and, therefore, its revenue and that was something the company was prepared to fight hard to retain. An objection to the licence was lodged with the licensing board and an enquiry was held. To the dismay of the smaller airline, BOAC's objection was upheld and Cunard-Eagle's licence to operate across the Atlantic to New York was revoked.

The purchase of the two 707s had been a huge financial undertaking and to operate them on routes other than those for which they had been intended was not something for which Cunard-Eagle had been prepared. The North American route was the one route that would have enabled the company to recoup some of its outlay and without it Cunard-Eagle had little use for the

707s. It had been too late to cancel the order as the first aircraft had been delivered on 27 February 1962 and had been given the Bermudan registration, VR-BBW, since it was now planned to fly it on the route between London and Nassau via Bermuda. The licence for this route was held by Cunard-Eagle's Bermudan subsidiary which meant that the aircraft had to be registered there. Further plans were made to extend the service on to Montego Bay in Jamaica in the hope that it would become more profitable. The inaugural flight departed London on 5 May 1962 but because the service operated only twice weekly the aircraft was not fully utilized.

In the meantime BOAC and the Cunard Steamship company had been conducting secret negotiations. Cunard decided to end its agreement with Eagle and, on 6 June 1962, a new company, BOAC-Cunard, was formed with BOAC holding 70 per cent of the shares. This meant the end for Cunard-Eagle but Eagle itself continued to operate as British Eagle International Airways although it didn't take delivery of its second 707, allocated the registration VR-BBZ, which was never used. Instead it went direct to BOAC on 7 July and was given the registration G-ARWE – Whisky Echo. It was followed on 28 September by the other 707 which had been re-registered by BOAC as G-ARWD – Whisky Delta. Both aircraft were operated by BOAC on behalf of BOAC-Cunard but this partnership was eventually dissolved in 1966 and they were registered to BOAC on 12 October. Whisky Delta served with BOAC until the beginning of 1973 when it was leased to BEA Airtours (later British Airtours) and it ended its flying career in 1981. It was sold to the Boeing Aircraft Company and was scrapped in May of that year in Kingman, Arizona. Its sister aircraft, Whisky Echo, would not be so lucky.

Just over six months after it began its service with BOAC, Whisky Echo had its first minor accident when, in the freezing winter of 1962-3, it was hit by a loading vehicle which was reversing away from the rear hold, prior to the aircraft leaving Heathrow for a flight to New York. The ground was covered in ice and the driver, who had had a twenty-two year trouble-free career, could not stop the vehicle from sliding sideways and coming into contact with the trailing edge of the starboard outer flap. The accident caused a 2-inch dent but the aircraft was soon repaired.

In the six years that Whisky Echo flew for BOAC it, in common with all airliners and, indeed, other forms of transport, suffered other minor maintenance problems. These ranged from burst tyres after training flights at both Stansted and Shannon; the malfunctioning of a light indicating whether or not the undercarriage was locked in place on a flight from Caracas to Bogota; a cracked window on a flight between Frankfurt and Beirut; a bird strike on a flight from London to New York and the occasional knock from a loading vehicle, catering truck or refuelling bowser in places such as Montreal, New York, Darwin and Sydney.

In Montreal, in the summer of 1966, while Whisky Echo was parked at Gate 33, the jet efflux from an Air France 707 blew a jeep which was parked nearby, into the port side of the aircraft, holing it in two places. The remainder of the flight was cancelled and the aircraft was taken out of service while the damage was repaired. There were one or two instances where the engine compressor blades failed, which led Rolls-Royce, the manufacturers of the aircraft's Conway 508 engines, to amend the maintenance manuals, and to introduce grit blasting of the blade roots to improve the fatigue life of the blades themselves. It is a tribute to the thoroughness of BOAC and its engineering staff that every incident was meticulously logged and investigated, and that not only were excellent repairs made but the lessons that were learnt from the incidents, in some cases, led to changes in procedures and policy that would ensure greater safety for the airline industry as a whole.

During the last year of Whisky Echo's life there were three incidents, one of which was very similar to the accident that destroyed the aircraft in 1968.

The first happened in Frankfurt in early May 1967 on a flight which had begun in Sydney. The stop before Frankfurt had been Rome and the aircraft arrived from the Italian capital at 09.41 on a bright clear morning, and parked at Stand 6. After the usual checks, refuelling and boarding of passengers, the doors were closed, clearance was sought and given for the starting of engines and the First Officer began taxiing the aircraft to the holding point for runway 25R. The charts which showed the parking positions at Frankfurt-am-Main airport gave recommendations as to where to turn to position for runway 07 but there was no similar advice for runway 25R. Worse still the chart for Ground Movement Control and Start-up Procedures did not have any of the positions of the stands marked, and showed the holding point for runway 25R as being where Stand 1 had been built. The First Officer had to decide for himself how to get to the holding point for runway 25R and elected to turn right and proceed through the area of Stand 1. Unfortunately he misjudged the distance and angle of the turn and the port wingtip hit the passenger loading bridge on Stand 1. The yellow guide line through the stand, which should have indicated the central position, allowed a mere 18 feet clearance between the loading bridge and the 707's wingtip. In addition the 142 feet 5 inch wingspan of the aircraft and the sweep of the wings made tight turns difficult and, on further investigation, it was discovered that the guide line was not in a central position anyway and there were other lines on the tarmac which were obsolete and misleading but had not been obliterated when the stand had been built.

The flight had to be cancelled. The passengers were rebooked on other flights to London and the aircraft had a new wingtip fitted and a temporary repair made to the wing's leading edge. It was ferried back to Heathrow by the crew, and major repairs were carried out at the airline's maintenance base. Although BOAC acknowledged that their procedure for updating the airport charts needed improving, it was also felt that the Frankfurt airport authorities needed to ensure that the ground markings were accurate and did not mislead pilots.

Just over six months later came what was the most serious incident Whisky Echo had suffered up to that point in its life with BOAC.

At lunchtime on 21 November the aircraft was preparing to leave Honolulu for Tokyo. It was a hot, clear day with visibility of fifteen miles as the 707 began its take-off run. As it reached a speed of just over 100 knots the No. 4 engine LP1 turbine rim and blading, and the Nos. 1 and 2 turbine stators broke off and smashed through the engine casing. The debris from the engine holed the wing and fuselage and the Nos. 2, 3 and 4 rear main wheel tyres. The thrust reverser unit in No. 4 engine also broke away and fuel began leaking from the damaged wing. It rapidly ignited in the jet efflux from the engine but because the aircraft had not yet reached the point of no return in its take-off run the crew were able to abandon the take-off. As the aircraft decelerated there were two explosions heard and a fire in No. 4 engine broke out. This was reported by air traffic control to the crew who immediately carried out an engine shut down drill. The fact of the fire explained the observation of the Flight Engineer that '...all No. 4 instruments were haywire'.

When questioned the Captain said that at around 100 knots he had heard a loud explosion and the aircraft began shaking. He immediately decided to abandon take-off but at this point neither he nor the rest of the cockpit crew were aware that the aircraft was on fire. Having made the decision to stop, the Captain then discovered that he had a problem with the thrust reverser on No. 4 engine because the lever was jammed open about one third. He applied full reverse on the inboard engines and corrected the resultant swing to starboard. He then made a rapid turn onto a taxiway where the aircraft came to a stop. The remaining engines were shut down, electrics switched off and an evacuation of the aircraft was ordered by the Captain.

Since No. 4 is the outboard engine on the starboard wing, the evacuation had to take place via the port side of the aircraft and a steward at the forward port door immediately opened it and tried to deploy the chute. Something went wrong with it, however, and it began to inflate within its container in the cabin. Having done so it ripped and deflated and was of no further use.

The fire was, by now, being brought under control by the Honolulu airport fire service but, when a stewardess opened the starboard over-wing emergency exit, smoke and foam poured into the cabin. The port over-wing exit was opened and some passengers escaped through this but six were injured doing so.

The remaining passengers and crew all left the aircraft via the port rear door where the chute functioned perfectly. None of the passengers received life-threatening injuries and those that were hurt were given medical attention at the Hickam Air Force Base Dispensary. Two passengers with broken bones were taken on to the Queen's Hospital so that X-rays could be taken and, in the case of one woman, for an operation on a broken ankle the following day.

During the enquiry into the accident it was revealed that the malfunctioning chute had been incorrectly deployed. The release drill was a two-part operation. When the container housing the chute had been opened the chute had to be rigged and a rip cord pulled to release it from the container. Having done this the chute was thrown out of the door and the air bottle discharge release handle pulled to inflate it. The enquiry revealed that the steward had forgotten to pull the rip cord and so when the air bottle handle was pulled the chute inflated within the container until the increasing pressure of the air caused it to burst out of the container and rupture. The bottom pin of the rip cord assembly and all the centre fastener eyelets were bent, with three of the fasteners having been torn away completely. With the fasteners bent and broken it was possible to push the chute out of the aircraft but the one foot tear in its underside, about one third of its length from the bottom, rendered it completely unusable.

When the surface of the runway was inspected two days after the accident it was found to be pitted and the shape of the marks was consistent with impact from turbine blades. There were turbine blades on and to the side of the runway and the thrust reverser that had broken away from No. 4 engine was found 50 feet from the right-hand edge of the runway and 3,250 feet from its threshold.

The No. 4 engine was actually older than the aircraft itself, having been manufactured in February 1960. Its total service time up to this point had been 16,280 hours but it had had a major overhaul at BOAC's Engine Overhaul facility at Treforest in south Wales three and a half months before the accident. It had then been sent to Delhi as a spare and was fitted to Whisky

Echo on 30 August 1967. It had since flown for only 868 hours. At the overhaul the main thrust bearing had been replaced by a new one which had a new modification standard and introduced a modified cage and vacuum melted balls and races.

Following the accident the engine was recovered and sent to Rolls-Royce in Derby who carried out an inspection on 6 December 1967 and confirmed that the main thrust bearing had failed. It was believed that the failure had been caused by a fracture to one of the balls. BOAC immediately recalled all engines fitted with bearings to this standard and a new modification was issued with the work on all the affected engines planned to have been completed by the end of June 1968. The enquiry made by the airline suggested that the fire damage was greater than it should have been because it was likely that the first officer had pressed the wrong button on the fire bottle to extinguish the blaze and when the flight engineer tried to correct this mistake nothing happened because, by then, the power had been switched off completely during the engine shutdown drill. BOAC decided to amend the flight manuals and emergency check lists as a result of this incident to ensure it could not happen again.

The steward who had not been able to deploy the chute properly was sent for additional training and it was decided, as a result of this accident, to review the training procedures for using chutes, to ensure that all cabin crew had hands-on experience. Until this time it was usual for stewards to open doors, and deploy chutes when necessary. Stewardesses were instructed on the theory of the operation but, in practice, never touched either doors or chutes unless they worked with stewards who would allow them some practice.

Accidents to aircraft can come in all different forms and, on 1 March 1968, Whisky Echo was involved in an incident that, had it not been for the quick thinking of an air traffic controller and the BOAC pilot, could have been a disaster.

The aircraft was making a scheduled flight from New York's Kennedy airport to Heathrow on a clear but windy day. Behind Whisky Echo a Pan Am 707 was waiting to take off and 9,000 feet from the threshold of the runway a de Havilland Twin Otter belonging to the commuter operator, Pilgrim Airlines of Groton, Connecticut, was waiting on a taxiway for clearance to turn onto the runway for its departure. The runway surface was wet as Whisky Echo, operating that day as flight BA 530, was cleared for take-off at 1634:35 GMT.

Five seconds after it began its take-off run the controller called up the Pan Am aircraft, flight PA 100, and positioned it ready for its departure. Thirty seconds after Whisky Echo confirmed it was rolling the controller calmly announced 'Ah Speedbird 530 abort your take-off'. Whisky Echo was at this point hurtling down the runway at a speed of 123 knots and was 7,500 feet from the runway threshold. The reason for this abrupt order was that the Pilgrim Airlines crew, despite being able to hear all the instructions to the other aircraft, had decided to position themselves ready for their departure and were, at this point, turning onto the runway a mere 1,500 feet from where the BOAC 707 was bearing down upon them at great speed.

The BOAC crew managed to stop Whisky Echo and taxied it off the runway where it was met by the fire services who checked the brakes, which were extremely hot but judged to be safe. The aircraft was then taxied back to the ramp and the passengers were disembarked so that further maintenance checks could be made. Meanwhile the controller was attempting to find out what the Pilgrim Airlines crew thought it was doing. The pilot of the small aircraft seemed to be totally oblivious to the fact that not only had he endangered another aircraft, he had put himself, his aircraft and its passengers in a position where, but for the quick thinking of the controller and the skill of the BOAC pilot, they would all, almost certainly, have been killed. When the controller called him up and asked, 'Who put you into position?' he was still unaware that he had done anything wrong and simply replied, 'Oh, we're in position and holding Sir' to which the controller countered, 'Negative clear the runway immediately'. Only then did he appear to realize that all was not well as he answered, 'Oh, ah roger'.

The last three incidents to happen to Whisky Echo before the one which destroyed it, give some idea of the causes and combinations of reasons that produce accidents. It is very rare that there is just one reason for a bad accident. It is usually a whole range of circumstances that combine to create the incident.

In the case of the first accident in Frankfurt the charts were found to be out of date, the most experienced of the pilots was not in charge of the aircraft at the point it hit the air bridge and the airport authorities had not ensured that the ground markings were clear and correct. In Honolulu, the most serious of the three incidents, the cause was due to a failure of an engine part which, having failed, went on to damage other engine parts and cause a fire to take hold. Had the fire bottles been deployed correctly the damage could have been limited but in both these cases the airline used the lessons it had learned to improve its safety standards as a whole.

The near miss on the runway at Kennedy airport shows that however good an airline's procedures and safety standards might be, outside actions and circumstances sometime create accidents that simply cannot be avoided. If Whisky Echo had been further into its take-off run when the Pilgrim Airlines Twin Otter started to turn onto the runway the chances of the crew being able to abort the take-off would have been almost non-existent.

Although airlines can and do take steps to improve methods of operation, there is very little that can be done to guarantee that a moment of distraction or a lack of concentration can be avoided and errors by anyone who works on an aircraft, on the ground or in the air, will always be the weak spot in the pursuit of greater safety.

Chapter 3

The Final Briefing

Having left their schooldays behind, the four members of the little gang from Scarborough Girls High School began to meet new people and change the direction in which their lives were heading.

Although she had become a civil servant upon leaving school, Kay still wanted to be an air hostess and was planning to apply to an airline. In 1964 Sheila married her boyfriend, John, and asked Jane to be her bridesmaid. She happily agreed and, later on, when Sheila had her children, Jane became godmother to one of them.

Margaret left the Halifax Building Society and, in 1967, moved to Rome where she had obtained a position with the United Nations Food and Agriculture Organization.

Jane, too, was beginning to reconsider her choice of career. Although she liked her job at the bank it was a little bit dull for a lively teenager and, having heard Kay speak of her desire to become an air hostess Jane began to think that this might also be something she would enjoy. She certainly liked travelling and she had the sort of personality that would be ideal for a job caring for passengers' needs and safety. She decided to apply to BOAC but, when she discovered that she was too young to be considered, began to plan how she would gain enough relevant experience to ensure that the airline would take her on once she was old enough.

In the 1960s when air travel was something experienced by a minority rather than the majority that it is today, obtaining a position as an air hostess, or stewardess as they were known in BOAC, was not an easy task. Girls had to be twenty-one years old, single, with experience of nursing or child care and able to speak a second or even third language with a good level of fluency. Prospective stewardesses had to attend a selection process which often involved more than one interview and which could take several weeks or even months to complete. Standards were extremely high and the offer of an initial interview in no way guaranteed the interviewee a position.

Stewardesses are often regarded by members of the public as decorative mile-high waitresses whose prime aim in getting the job is to meet and marry either a pilot or a rich passenger. There may be some whose intentions are exactly that but being a stewardess, especially in the 1960s, was so much more than pouring cups of coffee or chatting up eligible bachelors. Prospective stewardesses had to be pleasant and smart in appearance, especially as they would be wearing a uniform and would, therefore, be a symbol of the airline itself. They had to be personable but not over friendly, capable of dealing with difficult or demanding passengers without losing their tempers, and calm and decisive in a crisis. If there was an element of waitressing in the job it was silver service rather than transport cafe standards that were required.

Despite popular belief, the main function of a cabin crew member, male or female, is to ensure the comfort and safety of the passengers. In 1986 in a paper on Passenger Cabin Safety for The Royal Aeronautical Society, Dr R.B. Maclaren, then Senior Medical Officer at British Airways, outlined the cabin crew duties:

> In commercial air transport operations the role of cabin crew may be described as assisting in the provision of rapid, comfortable and safe travel through an environment that is potentially hostile and occasionally lethal.

He explained that:

> In the United Kingdom the Air Navigation Order requires that every member of the crew engaged on a flight for the purpose of public transport shall have been tested by, or on behalf of the operator and shall have practised their

knowledge and practical abilities in the use of emergency and life saving equipment. ...Training must be given in First Aid and in the use of appropriate equipment on the aircraft, in the use of therapeutic and emergency oxygen supplies and, most particularly, in dealing with emergency situations involving fire and smoke in the cabin: this latter to include passenger awareness of special hazards and checking of areas at risk; the proper selection and use of extinguishing agents; the role of ground emergency services and coordination with these in the need of emergency evacuation; crowd control techniques and the effective use of communications and demonstration of the problems of fire fighting specific to aircraft cabin conditions.

When one considers these aims, the additional requirements for the serving of meals and refreshments seem insignificant.

Jane Harrison had all the personal qualities required to become a stewardess. She was gregarious, well travelled herself, so used to mixing with different nationalities, and she had a caring nature. Although the photo of her in her BOAC uniform, when she was finally accepted as a stewardess, shows a neat, tidy young woman with a slight smile, it is a rather formal picture and doesn't do credit to the laughing, pretty girl with twinkling eyes that can be seen in all her other, more personal photos. Her housekeeping skills left a lot to be desired but airline meals were pre-cooked and just had to be heated so this small flaw would not put a stop to her plans. She did recognize that she needed to improve her language skills and decided that the best way to do that would be to live and work abroad for a few months.

Jane's cousin, Patrick Worthington, had married and was living in Switzerland at this time and Jane asked if he would help her obtain a position as a nanny in Switzerland so that she could improve her French. Patrick was pleased to help and put an advertisement in a newspaper for her. He received several replies from people interested in having a young English nanny for their children. Most were from families from the town of La Chaux de Fonds in the canton of Neuchâtel, where Patrick lived. The Art Deco architect Le Corbusier, famous for many buildings including the UN building in New York, was a native of the town, and its main industry was watch making, being the home of such renowned watch makers as Breitling and Tag Heuer; it would have been an ideal place for Jane to work and to improve her French. Had she chosen to accept one of the offers of employment from a family in the town she would also have had a ready made social life as it offered cafes, music clubs, cinemas and dancing, as well as parks and museums. Instead she chose to respond to the reply from a farmer who lived miles away from La Chaux de Fonds in what was the coldest valley in Switzerland.

The farmer, Monsieur Giroud, had two daughters aged eight and ten and Jane not only had to look after them, she had to be the first one up in the morning to light the fires in the house, before helping the farmer himself, which often entailed driving the jeep or riding a horse. Her experience of driving a jeep was non-existent; at this point she didn't even have a driving licence and she had an accident, fortunately not too serious, when she skidded off the road and ended up in a deep snowdrift. Although she had done some horse riding it wasn't anything like that which was expected of her on the farm. This was hard riding over hedges and banks and in deep snow. Once she fell off the horse and it rolled on top of her. She told her cousin's wife that she had been very frightened but she did not want M. Giroud to know.

She did have some time to herself each weekend when she would go skating on a frozen lake but if she wanted to go into town she had to catch a bus and it only operated every two hours so it wasn't a particularly easy journey.

Everyone on the farm liked Jane and when it came time for her to return to England they were all very sorry to see her go. The two little girls were in tears and didn't want her to leave at all.

Much later Patrick wrote a letter to Alan Harrison in which he said of Jane:

The very fact that she chose that farm shows something of her character. We had eleven replies to the advert we put in the paper and we warned her that the farm was miles from anywhere. …There are not many girls of her age who would have done the same.

Having returned to England Jane decided to work again as a nanny and contacted a company which was recruiting English girls to work in America. She flew out to San Francisco where she was placed with Dr and Mrs Allende and their daughter and son. Jane's job was to look after the boy who was called Jeffrey. The family lived in a large house and Jane had her own self-contained flat within the house, but it came with a price. Mrs Allende always expected her own needs and those of her family to come before Jane's and she often had to cancel any personal plans that she had made for what was supposed to be her free time. Although she had her own flat she preferred not to spend much time there on days off in case Mrs Allende found her something extra to do. Instead she and her English friend, Gloria, a housekeeper, preferred to go to the apartment of some other English girls who were working in San Francisco.

Dawn Bailey and her friends, sisters Irene and Margaret Akerstedt had been nannies on the east coast of America but, having finished their stint of childminding and obtained their US green cards, they moved to the west coast where they worked for a telephone company – Dawn and Margaret, or Margo as she was known, working in directory enquiries while Irene was in the international section. The three knew each other well as Dawn and Margo had been at school together before going to America. Dawn believes that they may have met Jane and her friend Gloria through another girl from Yorkshire who Irene knew from her work on the international switchboard. In different circumstances they may not have become friends; the main thing that they all had in common was that they were English but Dawn and Jane also had the shared desire to become stewardesses. Dawn, a year or two older than Jane, had discovered that her dream would not be fulfilled as her eyesight was not up to the exacting standards demanded by airlines then. Jane, however, applied to BOAC for a position while she was still in San Francisco. Dawn remembers her as having what she described as an 'assertive personality' – if Jane wanted something she went all out to get it – and Dawn believes that because of this she would have presented herself very well at her interview. It was Dawn, back in England for a holiday and recovering from chicken pox, who drove Jane to the interview with BOAC. She passed it with flying colours and began work with the company in May 1966, directly after her twenty-first birthday.

Jane's school friend Kay had also decided to become a nanny in America to gain experience that would be useful to her for her own application to an airline and had planned to join Jane on the west coast. Sadly for Kay it was at this time that Jane decided she had had enough of being the Allendes' nanny and made plans to visit her father's family, who were now living in Arizona, prior to returning to England. Since Kay didn't want to be in California without Jane she decided not to go after all. She stayed in Yorkshire and didn't pursue her dream of becoming a stewardess but remained in her civil service job.

The training that Jane received with BOAC was rigorous but she completed it successfully before becoming a crew member on the airline's Boeing 707 fleet. New stewards and stewardesses began their flying careers by working at the back of the aircraft in the economy class. It was hectic, hard work but Jane enjoyed it and loved visiting exotic places and meeting interesting and sometimes famous people. She wrote lots of postcards to her family and friends telling them about the places she had visited and the things she had done. When her cousin, Patrick, asked how she was coping with the non English speaking passengers, he found that she still lacked confidence in her ability to speak French. She told him that if she had a French speaking passenger she would pour him a large glass of whisky and then disappear down to the back of the aircraft and hide!

Working for BOAC had entailed a move to London and Jane left home and moved into a flat in Emperor's Gate, Kensington which she shared with some other BOAC stewardesses. She bought a car, a blue Ford Anglia, and used to drive herself to the airport when on duty. She was popular with her flatmates and they often spent their free time together. One of the photos in her album shows Jane and another girl sitting on a bed, smoking, with glasses of something, presumably alcoholic, in their hands. Jane captioned the photo 'Stewardesses Resting'. Despite having new friends and colleagues she didn't forget her old friends and kept in touch with her childhood companions too, writing letters and postcards to them all whenever she had a spare moment. She had boyfriends and had received at least one proposal of marriage which she had refused, saying that they were both still too young to settle down. She told her cousin Patrick that she had not yet met the man of her dreams.

Since she would be away for periods of up to three weeks or even more at a time, her free time after such a trip was generous and she, along with some of her colleagues, enrolled as a 'universal aunt'.

The company, Universal Aunts, was established in London in 1921 by a lady called Gertrude Maclean who had cared for numerous brothers, sisters, nieces and nephews before the First World War. After the war ended she found herself at a loose end until it was suggested that she could do for others what she had already done for her own family and the company was born. The Universal Aunts could be asked to do anything from house-keeping to gardening, taking care of elderly people or just plain babysitting. Many of the stewardesses who worked for the company in their spare time, including Jane, acted as babysitters when they were off duty in London. One of her assignments was to look after Jason Connery, son of Diane Cilento and her then husband, Sean Connery, while his parents attended a function. When they returned home Sean gave Jane a lift back to her flat in his Jensen Interceptor. She told her family all about it on one of the frequent postcards that she sent home.

Jane kept in touch with the girls she had met in San Francisco and when, in May 1967, Margo Akerstedt returned to London for her marriage to her American fiancé, Tony Sepe, Jane was invited to the wedding. Dawn was still in America and had not been able to get to London for the ceremony but Margo invited Dawn's parents in her place and also her cousin, Michael Moore, who had moved from his Welsh home to London and was living with his aunt and uncle. Michael, who was nine days older than Jane, worked very long shifts for the London Ambulance Service and had come to the reception directly from work. He

was sitting by the dance floor watching the festivities when Jane
spotted him and pulled him up from his seat to dance with her.
Later that evening when she said that she was leaving to get the
Tube back to South Kensington, Michael insisted on driving her
part of the way as he didn't like the idea of her travelling alone
in an area she didn't know. He had his uniform cap on the back
seat of his car and Jane put it on, asking if she could borrow it
so that she could pretend she was the pilot on her next flight.
Michael found her really easy to talk to. He said that she was
interested in what he was doing and was one of those rare
people who made you feel special when in her presence.
Michael enjoyed her company so much that he drove her all the
way home. Afterwards they remained in touch but met rarely
because of their work commitments. Today Michael still has
fond memories of the girl who made such an impression on him
that day and who he still describes as being 'a lovely person,
caring, bubbly and full of fun'.[1]

In the early part of 1968 Jane had a layover in Rome and was
able to spend some time with her friend, Margaret Jessop. It
was to be the last time they saw each other.

On 8 April 1968 Jane was rostered to work flight BA 712. She
drove herself to the airport and parked in the staff car park
where she met up with fellow stewardess, Rosalind Unwin.
They had not worked together before but chatted while they
waited for the BOAC bus to take them into the centre of the
airport to the Crew Reporting Office in Building 221. Jane told
Rosalind that she had particularly asked for this flight as she
had been invited to a wedding in Sydney. It was possible to put
in a bid for particular flights if one had a special reason for
wanting to be somewhere on a certain date and Jane was
pleased to have got the flight she had requested.

During the short bus journey Jane talked to Acting First
Officer John Hutchinson. He had worked for BOAC since
September 1966 but was already an experienced pilot, having
learnt to fly in the Royal Air Force. John had a pleasant chat
with Jane. She had just bought a new radio which she showed
to him and he said she was very pleased with it.

The pilot who would take flight 712 on the first sector of its journey to Sydney that day was forty-seven year old Captain Charles Wilson Ratcliffe Taylor, known to all as Cliff Taylor; the aircraft he would be flying was a Boeing 707 with the registration G-ARWE – Whisky Echo.

Cliff Taylor was, by birth, a New Zealander who had come to England in 1937 and had joined the Royal Air Force as an apprentice engineer, stationed at RAF Halton in Buckinghamshire. As a teenager his first love had been golf and, until he discovered flying, his ambition had been to be a golf professional. His plans were changed by the start of the Second World War when he retrained as a pilot, flying in Coastal Command throughout the hostilities.

Following his demobilization he joined BOAC where he flew a number of different types of aircraft including the world's first jet airliner, the Comet.

Cliff and his English wife, Audrey, had married in 1941 and had two daughters. He was a quiet, private man who enjoyed his family life, his home and his dog. Over the years the family had had a number of different dogs but in 1968 his pet was a black Labrador called Dinah. On 8 April Captain Taylor was driven to Heathrow from his home in Kent by his wife who dropped him off at the Crew Reporting Office and then set off for home herself. She wasn't expecting to see him again for another three weeks.

Cliff Taylor was a very experienced pilot. His total flying hours amounted to 14,878 of which 1,555 – the equivalent of nearly sixty-five continuous days and nights – had been spent flying 707s. However, whether a pilot had a small or a very large amount of experience, he was always subject to regular checks of his performance and capabilities, and it was Cliff Taylor's turn again on flight 712 when he was due to be monitored on the first leg to Zurich by fifty year old Check Captain, Geoffrey Sydney Moss who had been a supervisory captain on 707 aircraft for five years and whose own total flying experience amounted to 12,957 hours. A check captain's presence onboard an aircraft is to ensure that the airline's standards of operation are carried out by the pilot, not to take over any decision making, and he is expected to take no part in the workload of the crew, merely acting as an observer of the way the flight is conducted. Geoff Moss's presence on this flight meant that John Hutchinson, who would normally have been sitting in the jump seat behind Cliff Taylor, had to sit in the navigator's position. Captain Taylor usually briefed his third pilot to keep watch for any irregular occurrences in the cockpit and to monitor the outside of the aircraft through the cockpit windows. Since the check captain would be directly behind him in order to monitor his performance Cliff Taylor briefed him to also take the role that would normally have been that of John Hutchinson. John himself had very little to do on this leg of the journey as he was not in a position to be able to see clearly what was happening either at the front of the cockpit or on the outside.

Sitting in the right-hand seat, next to Cliff Taylor, was the thirty-two year old First Officer, Francis Brendan Kirkland and behind him was Flight Engineer Thomas Charles Hicks, aged thirty-five.

John Hutchinson's wife, Sue, and their two sons, were disappointed that John had to take the flight that day. He had spent the previous two weeks off and would now be away for three weeks just at the time of the boys' Easter holidays. As he left their Hertfordshire home that morning to go to Heathrow he bumped into his neighbour and spent a moment chatting to her and telling her where he was off to. He was carrying a fragile parcel with him that Sue had packed for a friend who was now living in Australia and who had been feeling homesick. Sue wanted her to have some familiar things from home and had packed a tray of new laid eggs from a local farm and two jars of homemade marmalade for John to deliver to her when he reached Sydney. When he got onboard Whisky Echo, John managed to slide the package under his seat where he thought it would be safe.

In addition to the five crew members in the cockpit there were six in the cabin. In the front, looking after the first class passengers were Andrew McCarthy and Rosalind Unwin; at the back attending to the economy class passengers were Bryan Taylor and Jane Harrison. The cabin crew was completed by Indian Stewardess Jennifer Suares and Chief Steward Neville Davis-Gordon.

Steward Andrew McCarthy had joined BOAC in 1959. He was a perfectionist and expected the same dedication from those working with him but, in spite of his exacting standards, he was a very popular member of staff. He had not been rostered to work that day. In the morning he had been to the airport for a meeting and had just got home when the telephone rang. He was on standby and didn't really want to answer it in case he was being called out but his wife, Christina, an ex-stewardess herself, thought that he might be in trouble if he did not take the call and so answered it herself. Sure enough it was from BOAC and Andrew listened, with a sinking heart, to the news that the steward who had been due to operate flight BA 712 that day had been held up and so he was needed back at the airport to work the flight himself. In view of what happened just hours later, Christina was very sorry that she had insisted on answering the phone.

When he got to the Crew Reporting Office Andrew was pleased to find that he would be making the trip with Jane Harrison as he had worked with her on several previous occasions and, like Michael Moore, thought her to be 'a lovely girl'. He noticed that she was wearing a black wig that day but thought that her own dark hair was much nicer and told her so, adding that she should pack the wig in her suitcase at their first layover and not wear it again![2] Jane used to joke that her very dark hair and blue eyes were due to her Celtic heritage on her father's side of the family but her sister says that her hair was very dark because she sometimes dyed it!

Andrew believed that this trip would probably be the last they would take together as Jane had hinted that she was going to stop flying. Her friend Kay said that the long haul flights had begun to lose their appeal for her and that she was considering applying for a position as a ground hostess in Australia. She thought that this may have been because Jane had a boyfriend in Sydney who worked as a pilot for the Australian airline, Qantas. The new boyfriend may even have been the reason for her request to work this particular flight as no one seems to remember any of Jane's friends getting married in Australia around that time.

Twenty-four year old Rosalind Unwin, from Coventry, had been a children's nurse in Switzerland before becoming a BOAC stewardess in 1965 and moving to a flat in Belgravia. Three years later she had travelled all over the world earning herself the nickname '007 Girl' after she was photographed in a bikini coming out of the water at Waikiki beach in Honolulu. The photo was reminiscent of the publicity shots of Ursula Andress from the 1962 James Bond film *Dr No*, although the actress was carrying seashells as she emerged from the waves whereas Rosalind had flippers and a snorkel, having been skin diving. She had learnt to dive while on a stopover in Bermuda.

Bryan Taylor, the second steward, came originally from Luton and had been working with BOAC for around the same time as Jane.

It was BOAC's custom to have at least one stewardess who was a national of one of the places in which the aircraft had a transit stop and these special crew members wore their national dress instead of the usual navy blue suit and white blouse. Jennifer Suares, whose home base was Delhi, wore a beautiful turquoise silk sari for her uniform.

In charge of the entire cabin crew was thirty-nine year old Neville Davis-Gordon. A married man with a fourteen year old daughter, Carole, he had joined BOAC as a catering apprentice on 7 May 1945, the day before VE Day. Apart from two years and three months spent doing his National Service, he had been with BOAC ever since and had nearly twenty-one years of service with the company, working his way up to his senior position with his calm efficiency and his professional attitude to the job. Before flying on the Boeing 707 he had worked on a number of different aircraft including the Douglas Dakota, Handley Page Hermes, Avro York, Canadair DC4M Argonaut, Lockheed Constellation, Bristol Britannia and various flying boats.

Monday, 8 April 1968, had dawned clear and bright. In homes right across the country people were getting ready for work or making plans for what they would do that day. Since it was the week before Easter, children were on holiday and were anticipating a day of play, far removed from the rigours of school and homework.

A small number of people were making their last minute arrangements before travelling to Heathrow that afternoon. Some were workers employed by the many airlines which used the UK's main airport; others were employed by companies providing services for the airlines such as fuelling, cleaning and catering; a smaller number worked for Customs and Excise or the Immigration service, while others had jobs that ensured the safety and wellbeing of all who used the facilities – air traffic controllers, policemen, firemen, doctors and nurses.

When Heathrow airport opened on 1 January 1946 its first flight was an Avro Lancastrian of British South American Airways, departing for the Argentinian capital Buenos Aires. There were no terminal buildings and the facilities were very basic for staff, passengers and all the other services needed for an international airport. Ten years after its first flight, building was in progress for the main airport services and terminals, to be located in the centre of the airfield between the two main runways. On the north side of the airport, close to where the original control tower and first prefabricated buildings had been situated, it was planned to build a new fire station.

By April 1968 the fire station was in place and Heathrow had three passenger terminals – the Britannic, Europa and Oceanic buildings – rather than the one which had originally been intended. They were situated in the centre of the airport and accessed via a tunnel under one of the two main runways. Later that year Terminal One was opened and the Britannic building, which was at the right hand end of the Europa building, was absorbed into the larger terminal which was then renamed Terminal Two. Terminal One was home to the airlines operating domestic flights and to British European Airways' continental flights. Terminal Two housed the European airlines with flights to their home bases across Europe. The Oceanic building, which would later become Terminal Three, operated the long haul flights to Africa, America, the Far East, Australia and New

Zealand and the biggest airline to use this terminal was BOAC.

The Oceanic building had been designed by architect Frederick Gibberd, who was responsible for the design of the entire central area when the airport facilities were moved from the original site beside the Bath Road. It was built in 1961 of glass and marble and was 143 yards wide and over eighteen yards deep. It was regarded as being the most glamorous of the terminal buildings, probably because of the exotic destinations of the flights that operated from it and the fact that visitors sometimes managed to catch a glimpse of arriving or departing celebrities. The exterior of the building became familiar to many people the world over because of its part in the Richard Burton and Elizabeth Taylor film *The VIPS*, although the interior was somewhat different, as that shown in the film had been built at the film studio.[3] Getting to the airport with heavy luggage was not an easy task. The Piccadilly line underground station was still some years away and even the A1 bus, which later operated from Hounslow West station, did not come into being until August the following year. Passengers intending to fly from Heathrow had either to take an airline bus from one of the London terminals in Victoria or Kensington, a taxi, a London Transport bus with probably several changes required, or have friends or family bring them to the airport by car. The latter option was usually the most popular as, having dropped off the passengers, the well-wishers could then stand on the open terrace on the roof of the Queen's Building and watch the aircraft take off. The runway closest to the roof terrace was 05R and visitors had a really good view from the Queen's Building of the aircraft taking-off and landing.

As on most days, the passengers who would use the airport on 8 April had destinations all over the world and their reasons for travelling were many. Among these passengers was a small group travelling on the BOAC flight, BA 712, to Sydney, Australia, via Zurich, Tel Aviv, Tehran, Bombay (now Mumbai), Singapore and Perth. There were 115 people who came from many different countries and walks of life, booked on the flight. Among these were several holiday-makers, some teenagers who had finished school for Easter and were going to spend the holidays with their families overseas, a positioning BOAC VC10 crew, a couple making a mercy dash to the bedside of their injured son, another couple returning to Australia to see their granddaughter for the first time, an ambassador returning home, several families emigrating to Australia, a fugitive from justice and a famous pop star.

Helena and Dorothy Morcam Taylor of Mill Hill, were on their way to Tehran to begin a lecture tour of Iran. The elderly sisters always illustrated their geographical talks with their own photos and had packed all their camera equipment in their hand baggage. Retired primary school teacher, Miss Nelly Abbott, was also going to Tehran and, like the Morcom Taylor sisters, was taking her camera with her. She, however, had a cine camera as she intended to make a film of her entire visit. Another elderly lady, making the holiday trip of a lifetime, was seventy-five year old Miss Marjorie Russell who lived in Holland Park, Kensington, and who had been saving for a long time to fulfil her ambition to visit India. The routing of flight 712 was unique for BOAC in that it encompassed a transit stop in the Israeli capital, Tel Aviv, followed by a stop in the Iranian capital, Tehran, and was the only flight starting in the United Kingdom to link a Jewish and a Moslem state in this way.

Passenger Katriel Katz had been a cabinet secretary in more than one Israeli government and was the Israeli Consul General in New York before becoming Tel Aviv's ambassador to Moscow, a position he had held the year before, during the Six-Day War of June 1967. He was famously called to the Kremlin by Andrei Gromyko, the Soviet Foreign Minister, when it became clear that war would break out between Israel and the Arab states. The Soviets supported the Arabs and Gromyko wanted to register his country's distaste for what he described as the 'war frenzy' in Israel. Katz was outraged and retaliated by excitedly detailing the threats made against Israel by the Syrians and Egyptians. Gromyko is said to have told Katz: 'Do not let your emotions get the better of you.' The situation between the two countries rapidly worsened and Katz was finally expelled from the Soviet Union. Regardless of the diplomatic stalemate that the two countries had reached, Gromyko was right in what he said about Katz letting his emotions get the better of him. By the end of Monday 8 April 1968 Katz must have wished that he had heeded Andrei Gromyko's advice of the previous year and not been in such an excitable state when confronted with the dangerous personal situation that would face him that day.

Iranian student, Maryam Entekhavi, eighteen year old house captain at her convent school in Bideford, Devon, was on her way to Tehran for the Easter holidays while another convent girl, seventeen year old Francesca Hall from Maidenhead in Berkshire was flying out to visit her father, who worked for BOAC in Singapore.

One of the passengers, Esther Cohen, had arrived in London from Buenos Aires via Lisbon. The widow, born seventy years before in Safed, one of Israel's four holy cities, was returning to her home in Maaleh Hashichrur, Haifa. Mrs Cohen was unable to travel without a wheelchair and needed a lot of help at check in and in getting onto the aircraft. She had been attended by a nurse during her transit stop at Heathrow but, the nurse told the BOAC crew, she would not need any help once she was safely in her seat near to the back of the 707.

Mary Smith from Winterbourne near Bristol was also a widow. She had lost her husband, Alfred, the previous November after nearly thirty years of marriage. The couple had both worked for Bristol Siddeley Engines, which later became the Bristol engines division of Rolls-Royce, he in the management audit department and she in the development fabrication department where she was a typist. They had not had any children but fifty-one year old Mary had two brothers who lived in Australia. She had not seen them for twelve years and she decided to visit them. She was taken to Heathrow from her home by other family members who planned to wave goodbye to her from the viewing terrace on the Queen's Building but she was making the long air journey to Australia alone.

Richard Hamond was also travelling alone. A marine biologist, he was on his way to Sydney to take up a position with the Commonwealth Scientific and Industrial Research Organization. A keen photographer, Hamond, from the village of Morston in Norfolk, had his Exa II 35mm camera packed in his hand baggage.

Twenty-nine year old Eric Blower was travelling to Perth alone too, although not by choice. The week before he had been demobbed from the Royal Air Force where he had spent nine years in ground electronics. He had found a job with IAL – International Aeradio Ltd, a subsidiary of BOAC – and was flying out to Perth to begin work with the company. Although he was a married man with a small daughter he was travelling alone because IAL had a rule that all employees must serve a three month probationary period before their families were allowed to join them overseas. Eric's journey had started at 7 a.m. when he boarded a flight to Heathrow from his home city of Leeds. If all went well with the new job and he remained in Australia, he would not see his wife Rita and their two year old daughter, Nicola, until July, when they would be eligible to join him.

Canon Wilfrid Elliott Henn and his wife Gladys Georgina, who liked to be known as Georgina or Georgy, had just spent five years in England. Canon Henn had been the vicar in the small Devonshire village of Branscombe but was now travelling back to his home town, Perth, in Western Australia, from where he was to take up a position at Bunbury, just over 100 miles to the south of the state capital. The canon and his wife were also looking forward to seeing their granddaughter, Susan, the daughter of their only son, Basil and his wife, Daphne. Susan had been born in 1964 and although she was already three years old she had not yet met her grandparents.

There were several other Australians returning home after visits to the United Kingdom. These included Annie and Catherine Shearer. Catherine, who was believed to have been Annie's daughter, had been born in Thurso, Caithness, Scotland and had emigrated with her family to Australia where she lived in Brighton, a suburb of Adelaide, South Australia. The twenty-four year old was a school teacher. The deputy general manager of the Australian Broadcasting Corporation, Clement Semmler, who had been on a seven week business trip, was also booked to travel on flight 712 and was planning a one day stay in

Singapore for shopping, before going on to his final destination which was Sydney. Lynaire Williamson was returning to her home in Hamilton, New Zealand, having spent the past three years working as a secretary in London. Her travelling companion was fellow New Zealander, Marion Bartlett.

William Rawson, an American from Annandale, Virginia, was making the trip to Tel Aviv on behalf of the American government. He worked for the National Science Foundation and was going to Israel to discuss three proposed government projects. Another American, Bill Deitsh, from New York was a Scientology lecturer and was travelling with fellow Scientologists, South Africans Alison Parkhouse of Cape Town and Brian Reso of Johannesburg.

Post Office telegraphist Stanley Thorpe and his wife, Grace, had come to Heathrow from Cherry Hinton in Cambridgeshire to take the flight as far as Perth where their son, twenty year old John, was lying unconscious in a hospital bed having had a motor cycle accident ten days before. When the news of the crash had reached his parents, the couple's friends had rallied round and raised £700 towards the cost of the tickets to Australia.

A thirty-three year old man from the north of England, had also reserved a seat on flight 712 that day. The father of four boys was intending to travel to Sydney and had booked his ticket with a travel agent in his home town. He told his family that he was going to Australia to look for work. A charge hand cable jointer, he was described by his father-in-law as: '...a jack-of-all-trades who could put his hand to anything'. However, the real reason for his unexpected trip to Australia, and one that was unknown to his family, was that he had been due to appear in the magistrates' court on the morning of 8 April, charged with indecently assaulting a fourteen year old girl. Rather than face a trial he had decided to flee the country.

Twenty-five year old pop singer, Mark Wynter, once described by Elvis Presley as 'one of your [Britain's] best new ballad boys', had a much better reason for taking flight 712 that day. Although he had a cabaret date to fulfil in a Melbourne hotel, his main purpose in going to Australia this time was for his wedding to his Australian fiancée, dancer Janeece Corlass. Since his first visit in 1961, Mark had been spending three months each year in Australia and had a huge number of fans there. During one of these visits Mark had met Janeece who was a ballet dancer on the Australian television channel GTV9. The wedding was to take place at 5 p.m. on Friday, 19 April after which Mark would fulfil the cabaret date at the Chevron Hotel in Melbourne before he and his new wife returned to England, having their delayed honeymoon in Italy on the way back. Mark was carrying his musical arrangements for the cabaret in his hand baggage and planned to go through them all at his leisure during the flight. In his cabin bag he also had a special fountain pen, engraved with his name, which had been his twenty-first birthday present from his fan club, and a small metal box containing his and Janeece's wedding rings. The new suit that he would be wearing for the marriage service was packed in his suitcase and checked into the aircraft hold.

There were twenty-four passengers on the flight who had made the life-changing decision to emigrate to Australia. Among them was young Steven Pragnell from St Mary Cray in Kent who was looking forward to his new life in Perth. The seven year old was travelling with his father, Fred – an electrical engineer – his mother, Vera, and his five year old sister, Dawn. The children were excited at the prospect of the long flight and the new life they were going to have. Fred Pragnell had only completed the sale of the family home some days before their departure and the family had spent their last morning in England at the home of a relative, where they took a final few photos in the garden. Holidays across the other side of the world were not usual in those days and they all knew that it might be many years before they saw each other again.

Perth was also the destination of the Molineaux family, John and Lilian and their children, Irene and John from Walworth, south London. The Hay family from Warsash near Southampton, was also going to live in Australia. Donald Hay and his wife, Patricia, had five children – Trevor, Diane, Kevin and twins Lorraine and Cheryl, and were the largest family to be emigrating on that flight. Fourteen year old Trevor was an ardent supporter of Southampton football club and had, in his cabin bag, his most prized possession – a complete set of autographs from the Saints.

There was another Southampton family, the Coopers, going to Perth to make a new life for themselves. Brian Cooper, his wife, Shirley, and their three children, Kevin, Jacqueline and Andrew, from Waterhouse Lane, Millbrook, in the south of the city, had been planning the move to Australia for some time. A month or so before they were due to leave England they had been watching a programme on television that showed a plane crash. Jacqueline who, like her mother and brothers, had never flown before, watched anxiously and said to her parents that she hoped that wouldn't happen to them. The pretty, blonde eight year old, a pupil of Foundry Lane School in Millbrook was, despite her delicate appearance, a real tomboy and if anyone dared to pick on her brother, Kevin, who was one year her senior, she would be the first to come to his assistance, delivering a good punch to would-be bullies. The brother and sister had a very close relationship. On 8 April the family arrived at Heathrow in plenty of time for their flight and were accompanied by a lot of family members who went up to the Queen's Building terrace to see them off. Before they left for Australia they too had time for a last family photo to be taken. It shows three well-dressed children – Jacqueline looking towards the camera with a slight smile on her face; Kevin and Andrew looking shyly down at the ground. The children's mother has a protective arm around the shoulder of her eldest child and their father squints slightly in the spring sunshine.

Air Traffic Control assistant, Frank Tyler, worked at the London Air Traffic Control Centre (LATCC) which was then located on the north side of Heathrow prior to its move to West Drayton in 1971. On 8 April he was rostered for a split shift – a morning and a night shift – and when he was getting ready for work he had put his 35mm camera in his bag, as he intended going up onto the roof terrace of the Queen's Building in between his shifts to photograph anything of interest that might arrive. One of Frank's colleagues, John Davis, had been a pilot in the Royal Air Force, flying Hawker Hunter jets before becoming an air traffic controller. On 8 April 1968 he arrived for his afternoon shift at 12.45 and, three quarters of an hour later, took up his position in the control tower.

Two and a half years before, John had been at work in Heathrow's control tower on a night blanketed in fog. In the early hours of the morning of 27 October 1965 a BEA Vickers Vanguard, G-APEE, carrying thirty passengers and six crew on a flight from Edinburgh, had made an ILS (instrument landing system) approach to runway 28R. The RVR (runway visual range) was only 400 metres and the fog was thick and swirling but it was still at a safe limit for landing. The first approach made by the Vanguard was unsuccessful and John then talked the aircraft down for an approach on runway 28L. This, too, resulted in another overshoot, and the aircraft flew off for a short distance to hold, pending another approach. This was made and was monitored by the PAR (precision approach radar) but resulted in another aborted landing. The aircraft started to climb away again but then made a steep dive and crashed onto the runway. For a few seconds there was confusion as, in the swirling fog, nothing could be seen. All that John and the other controllers knew was that there had been a terrific explosion but soon the night was lit with an eerie red glow as the aircraft was consumed in the resulting fire. All thirty-six people on board were killed in the accident. The enquiry into the cause of the crash, often referred to as the 'Double Echo' tragedy because of the aircraft's registration letters, laid much of the blame on the pilot who, it said, was tired and had had very little experience of overshooting or of landing in actual foggy conditions. It also cited the fact that the RVR lights were giving an inaccurate reading. Although John Davis was in no way to blame for the accident it was not a pleasant experience for him and was one he hoped would never happen to him again. It was the last thing on his mind as he began his work on 8 April.

Chapter 4

The Last Flight of Whisky Echo

Air travel was a much simpler affair in the 1960s than it is today. Passengers were asked to check in no later than one hour before departure and, in the days when terrorism was rare, there were no stringent security checks made. Baggage allowances were 66lb (30kg) for first class and 44lb (20kg) for economy which included the weight of the one piece of hand baggage passengers were allowed in the cabin, although most thought that this was extra to their checked baggage. Having presented themselves, their baggage, tickets, passports and vaccination certificates at the check-in desk downstairs in the Oceanic building, the passengers travelling on flight 712 were checked in, their baggage was tagged and sent off on conveyor belts to the baggage area behind the building to await loading onto the aircraft and they were given their boarding cards and asked to wait in the departure lounge upstairs. This was reached by going up the central main staircase in the terminal and through passport control which was directly in front of the stairs. Those passengers who were early or who wanted to prolong their last few moments with family or friends could have a drink in the Tavern in the Sky bar or a coffee at the snack bar. Once inside the departure lounge there was time to purchase duty free cigarettes and alcohol which then had to be carried on board the aircraft and stowed safely under one's seat along with the hand baggage. Overhead lockers were still in the future at this point and the racks above the seats could only be used to store hats, coats or blankets that would not injure anyone if they were to fall out during the flight.

The families travelling all the way to Australia would have

found it difficult to bring enough things to entertain their children in the hand baggage they were allowed, especially since the flight from London to Sydney would have taken around thirty-six hours, rather than the twenty-four hours, or less, that it does today. BOAC however, did carry comics and puzzles for their younger passengers and, in order to keep passengers, young and old, occupied, they served frequent meals, far more than was really necessary. There were no in-flight movies shown on BOAC aircraft in 1968.

While the passengers for flight BA 712 were being checked in, many other things were going on behind the scenes. The crew, both cockpit and cabin, were being briefed about the flight. The cockpit crew were given flight plans, fuel figures and meteorological details while the cabin crew received details about the number of people on board, the presence of any passengers requiring special attention such as Mrs Cohen, who needed a wheelchair, and any special meals that had been booked. The aircraft had been cleaned and fuelled, a departure gate had been allocated, the meals needed for the first leg to Zurich had been prepared and stowed on board and the ground engineers had made sure that there were no technical problems. A flight plan had been filed, cargo and mail had been checked and delivered, with its accompanying documents, to the aircraft side. A loading plan, telling the loaders where baggage, cargo and mail should be stored, had been handed to them and they had begun to put everything in its proper place in the hold. Later, when the check-in desks were closed and no more passengers were going to be accepted for the flight, the load sheet and the balance chart, detailing the weights and positions of cargo, mail, baggage and passengers, would be finalized ready for Cliff Taylor to check and add his signature to that of the dispatcher who brought the paperwork out to him in the cockpit just before departure time.

As on all flights, there was a lot of mail stowed onboard flight 712.

Doug Cotterell was a BOAC engineer, working for the airline in Singapore where he lived with his wife and two small boys. Every week Doug's mother, a teacher, would write a letter to her young grandsons, usually on a Sunday, and 7 April was no exception. She posted the letter that evening and it was delivered to Heathrow airport where it was loaded onto Whisky Echo the following day. Australian Diane Johnson,[1] who was living and working in London in 1968, wrote regularly to her mother in Sydney. She usually used a flimsy aerogramme but at the beginning of April had written a letter to send with some photos of her recent birthday. Her letter was also onboard Whisky Echo.

Included in the cargo for flight 712 was a consignment of what was known as 'dangerous goods'; items which, because of their nature, required special handling. These dangerous goods could be anything from poisons to corrosive substances or explosives. The dangerous consignment onboard Whisky Echo comprised 30 millicuries of Yttrium-90, a powerful beta-emitter – radioactive – which was being sent by the Isotope Production Unit at Harwell in Oxfordshire to the University Hospital in Jerusalem. Dangerous items such as this required very detailed documentation and careful handling and stowage on the aircraft to ensure the safety of the loaders, passengers and crew.

With one hour to go before the scheduled time of departure, the passengers for flight BA 712 were called to the gate. Those who would be travelling in first class boarded through the forward door on the port side of the aircraft and those booked in economy class through the rear port-side door. Many of the adults travelling on the flight, and most of the children, had not flown before and certainly not on a jet aircraft. It was a big adventure, especially for the children and one to which they had looked forward for some time.

As they walked to the departure gate Fred Pragnell remembers seeing a sign which read: 'Don't forget your insurance'. The sign was large, colourful and eye-catching but Fred ignored it and kept walking, without availing himself of the benefits it offered. Years later, when he and his wife returned to London for a holiday, Fred spotted the same sign. He pointed it out to Vera who said that she remembered it too but that it stood out so much more the first time they had seen it. They both thought how strange it was that it had seemed to leap out at them just before boarding Whisky Echo while later it was just an insignificant advertisement; one amongst many.

The passengers boarding Whisky Echo by the rear door were greeted by Bryan Taylor and Jane Harrison who showed them to their seats, which were upholstered in bold checked fabric in the latest BOAC style, and helped them stow their hand baggage and fasten their seat belts. Having helped the Pragnells find their seats and checked that their seat belts were correctly fastened, Jane leant across and asked the children, Steven and Dawn, if they had any friends or relatives at the airport seeing them off. She thought that they might be able to see them on the roof terrace if they did have anyone waving them off but Fred told her that they had travelled to Heathrow alone, fearing upsetting goodbyes at the airport and not wanting their relatives to have long journeys to get home. They settled back into their seats, to await the departure and relaxed to the sound of the soft music – *The Legend of the Glass Mountain* – that was playing in the background.

Soon all the passengers were seated and were looking forward to the first leg of their flight. Before they could leave, however, the cabin crew had to do the safety briefing, informing the passengers where the emergency exits were located, how to use oxygen should the emergency masks drop from the aircraft ceiling during the flight and what to do if the aircraft had to come down over water. They also pointed out that safety instruction cards were located in the seat pockets in front of each passenger. The seat pockets also contained in-flight magazines, postcards, and menus for the meal service the passengers could expect along the route, which usually provided a small diversion for bored, inquisitive children. As the cabin crew strapped themselves in for take-off they were already thinking of the afternoon tea service that they would begin as soon as the seatbelt sign had been switched off. Andrew McCarthy and Rosalind Unwin were at the front, just behind the cockpit in the jump seats by the door which faced towards the back of the aircraft; Jennifer Suares and Neville Davis-Gordon were sitting in seats 10D and 10E alongside the starboard overwing forward exit while Jane Harrison and Bryan Taylor were at the back of the cabin on the jump seats on the port side of the aircraft, facing forward.

With everything primed for departure, Whisky Echo was pushed back from its stand at 16.15 and started taxiing to the holding point ready for flight BA 712 to set off on its 13,000 mile journey to the other side of the world. Once it had reached the holding point the crew awaited instructions from the control tower to begin their take-off run. As the aircraft sat at the holding point waiting for clearance, Fred Pragnell thought he heard a muffled bang. He swears he did not imagine it and says:

> I spent most of my employment in testing electrical motors and generators, during which time I was tuned for unusual noises especially from machines.

Whatever it was that Fred heard, it was not noticed in the cockpit. John Hutchinson confirmed that everything at that point was working normally and that the cockpit crew had had no hint of what was about to happen.

John Davis, in the control tower, called up the crew in Whisky Echo and cleared the aircraft for line up and take-off but Captain Cliff Taylor told him they would need another two or three minutes before they were ready to go. He didn't say why the extra time was needed and John Davis assumed that it might have been to finish the safety briefing or ensure that all passengers were safely strapped in.

After the couple of minutes requested by the Captain had elapsed, the clearance was repeated from the tower and Whisky Echo moved to the end of the runway and immediately began its take-off run. The aircraft and the tower were in touch using VHF frequency 118.2 Mc/s – the same frequency used by all arriving and departing aircraft that day – so could be heard by the crews of all those aircraft.

The adult passengers relaxed as the aircraft sped along the runway while the children excitedly peered through the windows watching the airport seeming to vanish behind them in a blur. Then the aircraft became airborne. It left the ground at 16.27 and seconds later there was a loud bang and a violent lurch after which it continued climbing. What no one on board knew at that moment was that small parts of one of the engines had fallen from the aircraft and were lying on the ground at the end of runway 28L just inside the airport perimeter.

From his position in the control tower John Davis watched the aircraft as it left the runway and began a left turn. As it did so he saw what he thought was the late afternoon sun reflected on the port wing. He soon realized that it was not the sun but flames coming from one of the engines. Inside Whisky Echo's cabin some of the passengers had heard the bang and had seen the Chief Steward unfasten his seatbelt and quickly head for the cockpit. Andrew McCarthy got there before him and could tell by what he heard of the conversation between members of the cockpit crew that something serious had happened. The rest of the cabin crew were alert to the fact that all was not right but, at this point, the passengers didn't realize that they were about to experience the most harrowing few minutes of their lives. During the next few seconds many became aware of an increasingly serious problem.

Fred Pragnell noticed that:

> ... it didn't want to leave the ground. Up and down, up and down, until Vera said to me 'Look out the window, the engine's on fire'. I said 'don't be silly, it's probably burning off excess fuel'. Well, I was wrong. Vera mentioned it twice more and I had another look. I said, 'Shit, you're right'. I immediately turned round and told the steward [Bryan Taylor] to look out of his window. He was reluctant at first until I shouted, 'The engine's on fire'. He took one look and ran up through the cabin to the captain. I don't know what happened there but he came back and strapped himself in his seat.

Seventeen year old Irene Molineaux looked out of the window and saw flames. She turned to her father and told him that the plane was on fire. He apparently said, 'so it is',[2] and checked on his young son, John, making sure that the child's head was between his knees in the position that had just been demonstrated in the safety briefing.

Seated at the back of the aircraft American Bill Deitsh looked out of the window and said to his travelling companion, Alison Parkhouse, 'The engine is on fire'. She, thinking of the glow from the engines which can sometimes be seen at night, was unconcerned and merely replied, 'Doesn't that always happen?'[3]

On the ground fifteen year old Allan Blackman had taken advantage of the fine weather and the Easter break and had gone for a ride on his bike close to his home in Colnbrook, just to the west of Heathrow. As he cycled along, past the fields at the back of his house, he heard the roar of an aircraft which didn't sound quite right to him and looked up to see Whisky Echo with flames streaking out from the back of one of its engines. His bike didn't have any brakes and he nearly fell off as he tried to stop himself by dragging his feet on the ground. He yelled to two women who had stopped to have a chat along the road, 'Look, look! The plane...it's on fire!'

In the Poyle Trading Estate in Colnbrook, twenty-one year old Roy Stannett worked as a trainee draughtsman with a company called Graviner Manufacturing Ltd which was a part of the Wilkinson Sword Group. His office had a lot of windows and so offered a good view of aircraft taking-off and landing; a bonus for the young draughtsman who was an aircraft enthusiast. He recalled that:

The most impressive sights (and sounds) were witnessed on those occasions when the wind blew from an easterly direction, resulting in the landing aircraft, that were just seconds from touchdown, passing so low overhead that the registration marks beneath their wings could easily be read.

When the wind blew from a westerly direction, the direction of the prevailing winds, one enjoyed slightly less noise and a more distant view of the aircraft as they climbed out of Heathrow, having taken off from the southern runway 28L/10R, many turning south to fly over the Staines area while others continued their journey straight ahead in a westerly direction towards Windsor, Eton and Slough.

It was in just such conditions during the afternoon of 8 April that the normal flow of departures was punctuated by a distant but audible bang. Upon looking out of the window I was astonished to see a Boeing 707 trailing a long orange flame that appeared to stretch as far back as the aircraft's tail fin.

Roy thought it ironic that:

...among the company's many commercial safety products was a system known as FIREWIRE, an automatic detection system enabling both overheat and fire conditions in such locations as aircraft engines and fuel systems to be detected and, through the operation of cockpit controlled remote fire extinguishers, subsequently remedied whilst airborne.

From memory there was a tendency at this time for those aircraft in service with the principal British and Commonwealth airlines to be fitted with British airborne fire detection systems of Graviner manufacture. It is possible therefore that G-ARWE was fitted with such a system.

In Wraysbury, while Val Weir and her friend continued to follow the progress of the burning aircraft, seventeen year old Ewan Larcombe had also spotted it while he was walking past the Hythe End gravel pit. The flames coming from the back of the burning engine looked to him like an orange streamer and he ran along Staines Road until he reached the house of some friends and they all rushed up to a bedroom to get a better view of what was happening from the upstairs window.

By this time the passengers onboard Whisky Echo were now becoming aware that all was not right with the flight and were slowly realizing the seriousness of their situation. Mark Wynter, who was sitting in an aisle seat over the starboard wing looked across to the port side of the aircraft and saw what he, too, thought was the setting sun reflected on the wing. He soon realized, however, that it was not the sun but a fire, as he could see that the passengers sitting in the window seats on that side of the aircraft were beginning to lean towards the aisle. The fire was developing so quickly that its heat was starting to be felt inside the cabin. The man sitting next to Mark had previously told him that this was his first flight. He was naturally nervous about it anyway and, when he saw the fire, he began to cry. He was clearly terrified and Mark, an experienced traveller, tried to comfort him. It was a frightening experience for Mark too as, although he had flown many times before, he had never been on an aircraft that had a fire blazing on a wing only a few feet from where he was sitting. He had boarded the aircraft full of hope for the future – he had a very successful career and was about to get married – but now, suddenly, with the fire getting worse, nothing was certain anymore.

In the cockpit the crew was working frantically to find out what had happened and to keep Whisky Echo in the air. Having heard the bang and felt the vibrations it caused, the crew then saw the thrust lever for the No. 2 engine shift towards the closed position. Cliff Taylor ordered an Engine Failure Drill to be carried out and Flight Engineer Thomas Hicks began the drill at once. Because the undercarriage had already been retracted at this stage, the warning horn sounded when Hicks fully retarded the thrust lever on the crippled engine and both he and Check Captain Geoff Moss reached forward to pull the cancel switch and shut off the horn. At the same time First Officer Kirkland inadvertently hit the fire bell cancel switch which was in front of him. Thomas Hicks also reached for the engine fire shut-off handle but did not pull it as, at that time, no one in the cockpit was aware that there was a fire.

Geoff Moss's role in the cockpit that day was purely as an observer and his action in trying to shut off the warning horn must have been pure instinct. He left the operating crew to attend to their duties, turned in his seat to look back towards the port wing and let out a cry: 'Bloody hell! The wing's on fire!' Because the engines were slung in pods underneath the wing it was difficult for him to see the engine itself and he could only see the flames streaming back over the leading edge of the wing towards the rear of the aircraft.

In the control tower John Davis immediately instructed Cliff Taylor to turn downwind to keep the aircraft close to Heathrow for a landing on runway 28L, from which they had taken off only moments earlier. John could now see that not only was the engine on fire, the wing had flames coming from it too. He immediately hit the button to the crash line and declared an aircraft accident. His call informed the emergency services of the type of aircraft, where the accident had happened, or was likely to happen, and the rendezvous point for them to assemble to deal with the situation. At this point he could not even be sure that the crew would be able to nurse the aircraft through the air to make a landing at Heathrow at all, as the fire looked as if it was rapidly spreading.

As Whisky Echo continued its wide turn to the left it was seen by many more people on the ground. Seventeen year old Kevin Dent and his friend Graham had taken jobs during their Easter holidays and were working at Mayflower Nursery in Thorpe Lea Road which leads from Staines to the village of Thorpe. Kevin recalls someone rushing in to where he and Graham were working and shouting for them to come and look at an aircraft that was on fire. They ran outside and watched in horror as a large piece of burning wreckage fell off the 707 and plummeted to the ground no more than a mile or so from where they were standing. Sixteen year old Lesley Price was also working at the nursery during her school holiday and was busy deadheading carnations when she heard about the burning aircraft. She, too, rushed outside to look and saw the aircraft on fire but thinks that the engine had already fallen off at this point. On the edge of Thorpe Green ATCO John 'Tom' Toy had been standing outside the bungalow that he shared with several other controllers when he heard the aircraft approach. Being used to the regular traffic patterns, he was aware that the aircraft was in the wrong place and looked up. As he did so he also saw the burning wreckage fall out of the sky.

In Norlands Lane, Thorpe, several children were playing on the banks of a water-filled gravel pit belonging to Anthony de Marco of Marco Ltd, sand and gravel merchants. Mr de Marco himself was at the pit supervising the building of a bailey bridge and heard the aircraft approaching. As it made a slight turn he and the children saw the No. 2 engine fall from the wing into the gravel pit only fifty yards from where they were standing. It made an enormous splash and slowly sank into the gravel at the bottom of the thirty-feet deep pit. Police were soon on the spot

and questioned the children about the exact place that it had
entered the water. In the surrounding area small fragments of
wreckage were found in Egham, Englefield Green, Runnymede,
Thorpe, Chertsey and Stanwell Moor. Miraculously no one on
the ground was injured.

First Officer Francis Kirkland recalled that no one in the
cockpit was even aware that they had lost the number 2 engine
until after they had landed.

In Stanwell Moor on the south-eastern edge of the airport, nine
year old Keith Payne had been playing in his garden. An avid
plane spotter, Keith found it impossible to hear an aircraft and
not look up into the sky. As he heard the sound of Whisky
Echo's jet engines he looked up and saw a BOAC 707 in trouble.
Nearly forty years later and now an aircraft engineer himself, he
recalled:

> I can still see it today, glinting in the sunlight against a fea-
> tureless blue sky – with a bright orange fiery comet where
> the No. 2 nacelle should have been and the flames stretching
> back to halfway between the wing and tailplane. I stared at
> it as it tracked west over the house and backed into the
> garden so I would not lose sight of it behind the ridge tiles.
> It was shedding little black bits that looked like small pieces
> of black fabric but which I now realise must have been soot-
> blackened parts of the nacelle... .
>
> ...I was soon viewing it from the rear and then it started to
> roll left. For a second I thought I was about to see it roll
> inverted and go in but the roll stopped and, still burning and
> shedding bits, it commenced a gentle left turn. An orange
> fireball dropped and I thought 'Engine – the mountings have
> burnt through'... .

Back in Whisky Echo's cockpit the Engine Failure Drill had been
abandoned in favour of an Engine Fire Drill, a fact which was
relayed to the tower with the words from Cliff Taylor, 'Standby,
I have just carried out a fire drill'. None of the crew had heard
a fire warning bell, presumably because it had been shut off by

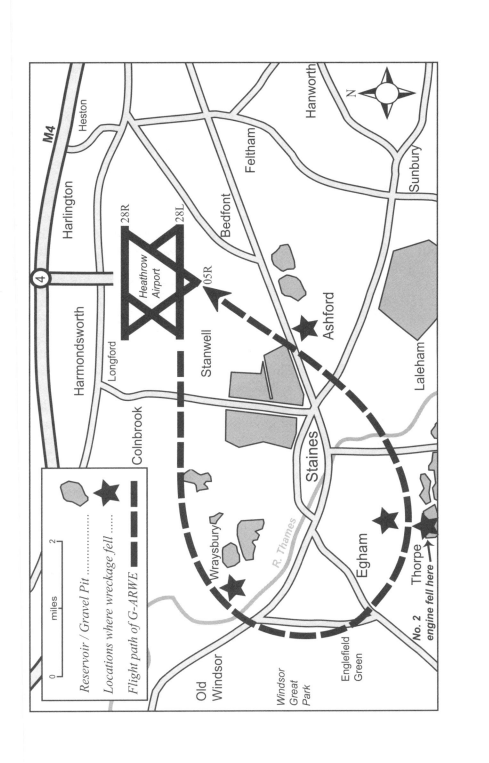

the First Officer, but the light on the No. 2 fire shut-off handle was on.

At a later date, and as a result of this accident, BOAC would change the procedures for the two drills – Engine Failure and Engine Fire – as the way they had to be carried out left a lot of scope for errors. The first part of each of the drills was done from memory and Thomas Hicks had quickly gone through Part 1 before reaching for his copy of the Part 2 checklist to complete the Fire Drill, which included operating the fire extinguisher transfer switch and also giving it another boost thirty seconds later. First Officer Kirkland had begun to read from his checklist but Thomas Hicks told him he had already done it so didn't continue.

Geoff Moss carried on monitoring the fire visually and reported that it was increasing, despite the extinguishers having been used. He told Cliff Taylor that he didn't think they had time to reach runway 28L and ordered him to land as quick as he possibly could. It was not within his remit to issue any orders on this flight, Cliff Taylor was the pilot in charge, but Geoff Moss could see what Captain Taylor could not, that the fire was now burning fiercely out of control, and the operating pilot took his advice and gave the tower another call declaring a Mayday and saying that he was coming in for a landing on any runway available. John Davis quickly responded. He still had the aircraft in sight and cleared it to land on runway 05R. This runway was hardly ever used and was significantly shorter than the two main runways. It didn't have any ILS facilities and had been built for the few occasions when there were crosswinds at Heathrow to enable aircraft to take-off and land into the wind. Although Whisky Echo's approach to this runway would signif-icantly reduce the remaining time in the air, the Captain would have to make a tight turn to line up for the landing and would have to stop as soon as possible to ensure that the overweight aircraft did not run off the end of the runway.

As Whisky Echo made its approach to Heathrow the ATCO hit the crash line once more to inform the emergency services where the aircraft was coming in to land so that they could be ready to assist when it came to a standstill. He also had to call up two other aircraft who were inbound into Heathrow and were heading for runway 28R to land. They were both instructed to overshoot and go round again as the two runways converged and John Davis couldn't be sure that Whisky Echo would be able to stop before reaching the end of 05R.

The way the airport had been constructed also created a problem for the emergency services as the police station and the main fire station were both situated on the north side of the airport and to reach the centre of the airport, in the quickest time possible, their vehicles would have to cross the live runway 28R rather than take the conventional route through the tunnel. There was a fire sub-station in the centre but its equipment was not sufficient to fight a large fire and most of the appliances came from the north side and had to get clearance from the control tower to cross over to the central area. This also applied to any other fire engines, ambulances and police cars that might be attending from forces outside the airport.

David Macdougald worked for Hall & Co., a concrete and cement company, at their base in Clockhouse Lane, Bedfont near to Heathrow. Just after 16.30 he was standing in the yard waiting for a delivery when he heard the sound of an aircraft. He thought that something was wrong with it but, at that moment, the telephone rang in the office and he went inside to answer it. The call came from his friend Dennis, who worked at the company's Chertsey plant and who had seen the engine fall from the aircraft very close to where he was standing. He told David to go back outside and watch the aircraft which, he said, was heading for Heathrow with smoke and flames pouring from its wing.

By now there were people in the streets, eyes turned skywards, in the entire area to the west and south of the airport. In Laleham Park across the River Thames from where the engine had fallen, fourteen year old Keith Harris was having an impromptu game of cricket with his friends. The match stopped abruptly as the teenagers watched in horror as pieces of the stricken jet fell off. Keith reflected that it had been a miracle that the engine had not fallen onto the densely populated caravan park to the south of Mixnams Lane near to where Thorpe Park theme park now stands.

From his garden in Thorpe Road, Egham Hythe, Malcolm Harvey watched the aircraft:

> I had gone inside to get my binoculars so could see every-
> thing clearly. The aircraft was not flying level; lots of
> sideways movement and this got worse after the engine fell
> off. This sight stays with me now and was probably the
> most frightening thing I've ever seen: like a dream, and I
> really did not think it would make it back to Heathrow.

As the cockpit crew worked frantically to bring the aircraft back home the cabin crew were preparing the passengers for an emergency landing and evacuation. Having just completed the safety briefing they walked up and down the aisle, again reminding passengers to remove their shoes, place their pillows on their laps, put their heads down on the pillows and keep their seatbelts fastened tightly.

From their seats in the second row of economy class, the elderly sisters, Dorothy and Helena Morcom Taylor, remem-bered seeing Chief Steward Neville Davis-Gordon disappear into the cockpit and then emerge seconds later to walk briskly down the aisle. When he was level with their seats he bent towards the sisters and said:

> Well, ladies, regretfully there is something wrong but
> nothing to worry about. Just put your pillows on your knees
> and put your head down on them and guard your face and
> tighten your seatbelt. We are going to make an emergency
> landing.[4]

His reassuring tone calmed their nerves and Helena Morcom Taylor commented to her sister that everything seemed to be 'beautifully under control'. Both ladies obeyed Neville Davis-Gordon's instructions. Some passengers were clutching the hands of their family members; others prayed. Mothers and fathers attended to their children, trying to keep them calm; somewhere in the cabin a baby cried.

The Cooper family was sitting at the back of the cabin. Brian and Shirley were with Andrew in one row but they had not been allocated adjoining seats when they checked in and Jacqueline and Kevin were two rows ahead of their parents and young brother. With the seatbelt sign still switched on, their parents could not get up to check that the two elder children were all right. Soon after take-off Shirley had looked out of the window and said to her husband: 'The engine is on fire.' He didn't believe it and replied: 'It can't be.' But he soon realized that it was.

Those passengers sitting on the port side of the cabin, especially those nearest to the wing, were the most vulnerable. They could see the flames spreading from the burning engine up and across the wing. Then they saw the engine mountings give way and the engine plummet to earth. The windows were so hot that they couldn't touch them and some were beginning to buckle as they started to melt. Although they had been told to remain in their seats, their instincts told them to move away from the source of the heat that was causing sweat to pour down their faces.

Fred Pragnell recalled that by this time the aircraft was:

...all over the place; people crying out. The cabin was bathed in an orange glow and small explosions could be heard. I was talking all the time to my wife and children telling them that the pilot up front knew what he was doing and that they should keep calm. I then said the Lord's Prayer and everything seemed to feel OK. The lady on my right was going to Australia to see her son in hospital in Sydney (I think he had a head injury). She was with her husband and she was gripping my right hand. Across the aisle my wife was gripping my left hand.

The noise was tremendous; the engines seemed to be making a hell of a noise. It seemed we were turning when all of a sudden the noise stopped, the plane gave a big lift up and suddenly a huge explosion took place. You could see pieces of wing coming off. I looked out of the window on one occasion and saw the cars driving along a highway and wondered where we were going to land.

Eric Blower had managed to get a window seat with two spare seats beside him. He was looking forward to the flight as, although he had flown before, this was his first flight in a jet aircraft and he was quite at ease as the aircraft left the ground on the start of its journey to Australia:

I suppose it was maybe 60 seconds or so later there was a loud crack/bang and the aircraft gave a slight bump. I thought that maybe it was some sort of turbulence but this caused me to focus my eyes onto the wing to my left, and it was then that I saw a small flame appear from the inside engine. I heard a man's voice shout 'my God, we are on fire'. The scene quickly changed from relative silence to lots of loud chatter with lots of 'ohs' and 'Gods' etc.

I remember thinking to myself that it was all some kind of dream or somehow that it was just not happening. Sadly it was happening, and very, very quickly that small flame had turned into what I can best describe to be like a gigantic blow lamp producing a deafening roar.

I haven't much sense of time from now on but very shortly after the crew sprang into action.

I remember the chief steward hurrying towards us from the front portion of the aircraft, (I remember his face was green), [he] shouted something about a problem and that we had to prepare for an emergency landing, (or something like that), and to put a cushion between our knees, bend forward and put our face into the cushion.

I think there was another steward and a stewardess in our part of the cabin at this time. I guess the stewardess was Jane Harrison but I'm not certain.

Whilst preparing to take up the emergency landing position I remember seeing the window close to me. It was becoming distorted, caused by the heat, which was now becoming overpowering.

I suppose now I was just waiting for the bang which, I was convinced, was going to come. I remember several explosions but not the big one, Not yet anyway.

Richard Hamond, the marine biologist, was sitting on the port side of the aircraft in seat number 19A, level with the trailing edge of the wing. When he had boarded the aircraft he had been disappointed to find that he didn't have a clear view from the window because of the wing but, having seen the fire which was blazing just a few feet away from where he sat, he decided that he would like to make a record of what was happening to the aircraft and the passengers and pulled out his camera to take some photos which he hoped would survive even if he did not. The light meter he used, started at level one and rose to level eighteen. When he began to take his photos, the level on the meter started to rise until eventually, when it was becoming too hot to focus the shots carefully, the level had risen to sixteen and Dr Hamond could not even look at the fire because the light was blinding him and the heat was intense.

Sitting next to him in seat 19B was fourteen year old Southampton football supporter Trevor Hay and, on his right, in seat 19C, was his brother, Kevin. In the row in front, in seats 18A and B were Trevor's mother, Patricia, and his sister Diane and, in front of them in seats 17A, B and C sat his father, Donald, and twin sisters, Lorraine and Cheryl. The entire family was in the worst possible position on the aircraft, directly next to where the fire was at its fiercest.

At the front of the cabin, stewardess Rosalind Unwin realized that they were in trouble and her anxiety increased when she saw the engine fall off the wing. Andrew McCarthy had also seen the engine fall but thought to himself, 'Good, it's missed us, now we have a chance'. Rosalind quickly made sure that the forward doorways were clear for the impending evacuation. She and Andrew had served drinks to the first class passengers before take-off and now she grabbed everything that they had used for that service and pushed it, along with her handbag, into one of the forward toilets to make sure that there were no obstacles for the passengers to fall over when the moment came for them to leave the burning aircraft. She then checked that the first class passengers were in the correct position for an emergency landing. She also spoke to the two members of the supernumerary VC10 crew, a captain and first officer, who were sitting in first class, and asked them to help with the evacuation.

They promised to do so although neither had worked on a Boeing 707 before and weren't confident that they would be of much help. Rosalind knew that she would do whatever it took to help get all the passengers off the aircraft but she also felt that she would be able to save herself too and never believed that she would die.

When Neville Davis-Gordon left his seat and hurried up to the cockpit, stewardess Jennifer Suares, who had been sitting next to him, glanced through a port window and saw the fire that was beginning to take hold of the engine and wing. She began to stand to attend to the passengers but also saw that the aircraft was flying very low and believed that they would not make it back to the airport but would crash on the way in. She changed her mind about comforting the passengers and instead began to demonstrate the emergency drill again just in case they remained airborne long enough to get back onto a runway and begin an evacuation. When the chief steward returned to his seat she grabbed a pillow for him to brace himself for the landing.

At the back of the aircraft Bryan Taylor and Jane were also checking that the doorways and aisle were clear and, having done so, sat down again in their seats and prepared themselves for a crash landing. They both knew by that stage that any evacuation from the rear of the aircraft would have to be done through the galley door on the starboard side, as the flames from the port wing were intensifying and would be far too close to the rear passenger door on that side for it to be a safe option. Fred Pragnell continued his story:

> Well, after the plane had turned and was diving down (we were previously told to prepare for a crash landing) I couldn't keep my head down and, as I said, I kept talking to the kids and anybody else if they wanted to listen, telling them that all is OK and that the pilot knew what he was doing, etc. I hoped it helped.
>
> It was getting very hot and people were crying out, obviously getting very close to getting burnt as by now it seemed that fuel was running down the left side of the plane; smoke was coming into the cabin. I remember thinking that

if my wife and kids are to get out I had better do something before everybody got out of their seats and came down to the back.

We were getting low now but pieces of the wing were still blowing off. There were also bright flashes. The plane was still all over the place and how that pilot managed to control it still amazes me when I look back on it. The fire trucks were now in view so I said to my wife, whose hand I was still holding, 'When we hit the runway don't undo the seatbelts until we hit a second time' (don't forget that I was cool, calm and at no time did I think we were going to get killed). The lady next to me was still holding my hand and was very distraught as you can imagine but I wanted to get up to make sure Vera could get herself and the children out of the seatbelts and out of their seats before the passage was blocked.

Although Fred had made sure that his family didn't undo their seat belts too early, he neglected to take his own advice and, as the aircraft hit the runway, he unbuckled his belt so as to be able to help his wife and children from their seats and was thrown upwards towards the roof before the aircraft finally settled down onto the ground. As he regained his footing he stood in the aisle and blocked the way to allow Vera and the children to leave their seats and get to the rear exit as quickly as possible. When he was sure that they were on their feet and moving towards the door he pushed in front of them to be able to help the children get out.

As he got to the rear exit he heard Jane and Bryan Taylor arguing about which of them would go down the aisle and help the passengers from their seats and direct them towards the emergency exits. He heard Jane say that it was her job and then Bryan saying he would do it. Fred asked them both whose job it was and Bryan confirmed that it was Jane's so Fred suggested that he should let her get on with it and that he should attend to his own responsibilities. Bryan had to be at the door as, not only was it the job of the steward to open the doors in an emergency, it was likely that Jane would not have been able to secure the chute, as the bars that held it in place were often very difficult to

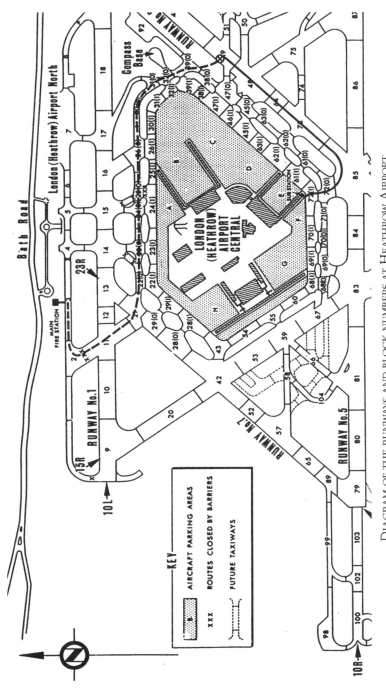

DIAGRAM OF THE RUNWAYS AND BLOCK NUMBERS AT HEATHROW AIRPORT.
WHISKY ECHO LANDED IN BLOCK 85 AND CAME TO REST IN BLOCK 49.

fit into their retaining clips and some element of force might be needed. The favoured method was a kick which would have been difficult for her to deliver when wearing stiletto heeled shoes. The securing of the chute did prove to be problematical and it was fortunate that Bryan had been stopped from taking over Jane's work and was on hand to use the force necessary to make the chute stable enough to be used.

In the final few seconds before landing, the friends and relatives who had gone to wave to their loved ones from the top of the Queen's Building as they started their journey to Australia, held their collective breath as they watched the fire damaged aircraft make its approach, and three minutes and thirty-two seconds after Whisky Echo took off from runway 28L Captain Taylor made a perfect emergency landing on runway 05R. Mark Wynter described it as like 'coming down in a lift'.

Air Traffic Control Assistant Frank Tyler was standing among the families on the viewing terrace of the Queen's Building. The aircraft touched down in block 85, the intersection with runway 28L and, as it slowed towards its final resting place in block 49, he took the dramatic photo that appears on the cover of this book.

The aircraft stopped abruptly and John Davis, in the tower, answered, in the affirmative, Cliff Taylor's call, asking for permission to disembark the passengers. The cabin crew hadn't waited for permission. They had already opened the doors while Whisky Echo was coming to a halt and had begun the evacuation the minute the aircraft was stationary.

Chapter 5

The Tragedy of Flight 712

Although runway 05R had been the only runway that gave the aircraft and its passengers any chance of survival, it did create its own problems. Cliff Taylor's landing had been a magnificent feat of airmanship. He had managed to bring the severely damaged 707 back to earth safely on three engines, well over its maximum landing weight and on a runway that was short, with no ILS and in a crosswind. Had there been more time, the ideal runway would have been the one from which Whisky Echo had taken off – aircraft both take-off and land into wind. The fact that 05R represented the only chance they had of surviving, meant that they had to land into a slight crosswind and, as the aircraft came to a stop, the flames that had been streaking out behind them suddenly changed direction as the light wind blew them from the port side of the aircraft towards the starboard side and the passengers' and crews' only escape route. The moment the aircraft was stationary the smoke that had been dissipated by the airflow, started to rise into the sky and all that the people in the surrounding areas could see was a huge thick black column which reached so high that it could be seen ten miles away.

After the calm, unflappable way he had dealt with the emergency and helped the aircraft to reach the ground safely, John Davis was dismayed when he looked out of the control tower window and saw nothing but a huge bonfire, burning out of control on the runway. He immediately began asking himself if there wasn't something else that he could have done to save the passengers and crew who, he now believed, had died in front of him. Had this been a normal shift he would have been due for a break by now anyway and, in view of the distressing experience he had just had, he was immediately relieved of his post and taken downstairs to the rest room where he was given a cup of tea. There he began to make notes of everything that had happened from the moment he had spoken to Whisky Echo before take-off until it disappeared from his sight in a cloud of acrid dense smoke on runway 05R.

Engineers working for British European Airways in the airline's maintenance buildings had also witnessed the landing of the burning aircraft. John Webb,[1] a licensed BEA charge hand who had been working for the airline for seventeen years spotted Whisky Echo:

> ...rolling along a runway apparently after landing. The port wing was on fire, the fire appeared quite intense but confined to the wing. With Mr. Jordan [a colleague] I left the building, climbed into a land rover and drove immediately towards the aircraft. We approached the aircraft from the port rear and I noticed that two fire appliances which had been following the aircraft down the runway were in position, one on the port side of the aircraft in line with the wing tip, the other immediately to the rear of the fin. The rear appliance was spraying the fin and the forward appliance was attacking the fire on the port wing. There was a very heavy fire in the port wing and in a lake of kerosene on the port side and under the centre section of the aircraft. I stopped the land rover some distance forward of the nose of the aircraft and noticed the front port door opened with probably an escape chute or rope dangling from the door, no one was visible at the door.

From the outside the situation looked very bad but, contrary to John Davis's belief, Whisky Echo hadn't become a huge funeral pyre. As soon as it reached block 49 and came to a stop Neville Davis-Gordon had opened both of the emergency exits over the starboard wing with the help of Flight Engineer Nev Boulton, one of the extra VC10 crew who had been sitting close by, and passengers started to get out onto the wing itself and then jump down to the runway below. The exits themselves were small and awkward to use as the passengers had to sit on the edge of the opening and bend their heads towards the floor while pulling up their feet. They were not much use for anyone who was overweight, and they required a degree of agility in order to be able to get through them. The chief steward calmly guided passengers towards the exits and ensured they had left their belongings behind in order to give themselves the best possible chance of survival. He was helped by Jennifer Suares who also directed passengers to the over-wing exits and helped them through. It was more difficult for her to move around the burning aircraft than it was for the other two stewardesses as she was still wearing her national dress.[2] Although a beautiful, graceful costume it was of no help in a situation such as the one onboard Whisky Echo. Later Neville Davis-Gordon said of his colleague:

> I must add that Miss Suares, with whom I worked during the emergency, was magnificent although hampered by the sari she has to wear.

Mark Wynter was one of the first passengers to escape through the over-wing exit. He had tried to take his hand baggage with him but Neville Davis-Gordon had stopped him, telling him he wouldn't need it and so it had been left behind when he climbed through the opening and leapt to

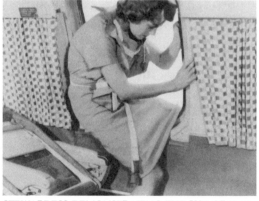

STEWARDESS DEMONSTRATING THE USE OF THE OVER-WING EMERGENCY EXIT OF A BOEING 707

safety. When he stood up he saw a girl wandering round, dazed, and put his arm around her shoulder and together they ran away from the aircraft and towards some buildings he estimated to be 200-300 yards away. As they ran, Mark heard several explosions and, when he turned to look back, saw that there were flames and smoke coming from all over the aircraft not just on the port side. He ran, as he says, 'like a lunatic' away from the inferno on 05R and only stopped when he and his companion reached the buildings. These turned out to be the offices and hangars of British Eagle, the airline which had once owned Whisky Echo, albeit very briefly, before BOAC had stepped in and taken it over, having successfully blocked the smaller airline's licence to operate across the Atlantic. Audrey Lendon, a secretary with British Eagle, remembered seeing the aircraft as it came down the runway past her office window, having landed just beyond the airline's administration block. She recalled that:

> By the time Eagle staff members came out of the buildings, the first of the passengers were coming off via chutes and then made their way along the taxiway to Eagle's base. Our Chairman's secretary and personal assistant Molly Gunn then brought the first of the passengers into the boardroom and offered refreshments.
>
> As further passengers came off they mainly congregated outside the hangars until the emergency services and police arrived.

Molly confirmed later that the refreshments offered involved opening the boardroom bar!

Eric Blower believes that at the moment he saw that the windows were beginning to melt he may have passed out briefly, but he cannot be sure. The next thing that he remembered was someone pushing or shaking his shoulder which, he says:

> ...kind of brought me round and a man's voice shouting, 'we are getting out'. I have never known who that person was. I just hope he knows what he did.

Eric then realized that, in those few seconds that are forever lost to him, the aircraft had landed:

We were on the ground. Passengers were in the aisle next to my seat and making towards a now opened emergency exit leading onto the starboard wing on the other side of the aircraft. I think the exit was two seats in front of mine. I remember the stewardess was supervising the evacuation, ordering us not to take anything with us and to leave our belongings behind. There was no panic, lots of noise and screams but no panicking.   Everything was indeed amazingly orderly. I stood up and made my way to this exit.

By now flames and smoke were everywhere, the smoke very thick and black. You couldn't see very much at all. I climbed out of the emergency exit onto the wing, shuffled very warily towards the edge of the wing (I couldn't see the edge) and jumped. Gladly it was painless. Survival mode then took over and immediately my feet touched the ground I just ran instinctively. It seemed like we were all running away from the aircraft and the rescue services and other airport staff were running towards the aircraft. I just remember running right into what appeared like a big man, his arms grabbing me and squeezing me into him. It was at that moment that there was an almighty bang. I turned round to look and the aircraft was barely recognisable. It was just a ball of flames.

At the front of the aircraft Rosalind Unwin had opened the forward door on the port side and was struggling to get the chute out of its container. When she pulled the rip chord to activate it, it broke off in her hand but she did eventually get the chute in place with help from Captain Taylor.

BEA engineering charge hand, Arnold Gosnold,[3] watching the scene from outside his office, heard an explosion which he thought was a fuel tank and saw that the centre section of the aircraft was enveloped in flames. He then saw the forward port door open and, what he took to be the escape chute being thrown out but noticed that it didn't seem to inflate. Following Rosalind's struggle with the chute at this door Thomas Hicks, the flight engineer, had climbed down to straighten it but before anyone could use it to make their escape, the fire that had intensified with the explosion of a fuel tank, set it alight and it was of no further use.

Andrew McCarthy had opened the forward starboard galley door but also had problems with the chute. The bar that, with the aid of retaining clips, was designed to hold the chute in place, was bent. Andrew managed to fix the problem by giving the bar a hefty kick with the heel of his shoe and it eventually fell into place. Rosalind moved to the galley door on the starboard side and helped Andrew get the majority of the passengers who used this exit, through the doorway and onto the chute. There was one elderly lady who refused to move and so Rosalind grabbed her by the neck and pushed her, kneeing her in the back until she fell onto the chute. Her assisted exit from the aircraft was completed by the next passenger to escape who pushed her in front of him as he slid down to the ground.

BEA engineer John Webb had, by this time, left his Land Rover and run around the front of the aircraft to the starboard side where he saw that the chute was beginning to be used by the passengers. He saw that:[4]

> There were about six people assisting at the bottom of the chute. Passengers at this time appeared to be in reasonable condition and I lent a hand in directing them away from the burning aircraft.

John Hutchinson and Cliff Taylor had come out of the cockpit and were helping Neville Davis-Gordon to get the passengers to the forward chute as quickly as possible. John commented that Neville gave orders in such a calm but forceful way that he was sure the passengers were more frightened of the Chief Steward than they were of the fire. The smoke from the back of the cabin was getting worse and the aircraft was lurching as the fire intensified. When the former ambassador, Katriel Katz, pushed his way to the front and tried to escape through the forward port door it was John Hutchinson and Rosalind Unwin who initially stopped him.[5] A large man, Katz was determined to use this door and, despite the crew's efforts to calm him and direct him to the safer forward exit on the opposite side of the 707, he would not listen to anyone and very nearly took Rosalind and

John with him as he broke free and leapt through the forward port doorway. Had he heeded the advice given to him the year before by Andrei Gromyko, and not been so hot-headed, he would undoubtedly have saved himself the many injuries he sustained when jumping onto the hard surface of the runway.

BEA aircraft handling officer, Charles Wiles,[6] who had driven out to the aircraft in a Land Rover to see if he could help, saw that the forward port over-wing exit was open but that no one was using it. He then saw:

> ...a passenger crawling and being dragged along the ground by another man in uniform from a position level with the over wing emergency exit. The uniformed man asked me to give him a hand. Between us we carried the injured man, who appeared to have badly damaged legs or ankle, to the land rover and took him to [the] BOAC medical centre.

Since Katriel Katz was the only passenger to leave the aircraft on the port side, it is probable that the man Charles Wiles helped was the Israeli diplomat. The fact that he saw him at a point that he estimated to be level with the wing's leading edge would seem to indicate that when he jumped, he not only hit the ground with some force but then rolled backwards on the runway, towards, not away, from the source of the fire.

Thirty-six year old BEA radio maintenance engineer, Douglas Jordan who had arrived at the scene with John Webb, noticed that someone was standing by the forward port door but that the chute was hanging, not inflated and useless.[7] He ran around to the starboard side and found a man lying injured in front of the aircraft's nose. He found another airport employee and together they managed to get the man to a safe distance from the aircraft. He then returned to find another man in an almost identical position and state:

> After about a minute I obtained the assistance of two other men and we carried the second injured man away from the aircraft. It appeared that his right leg or hip was broken; he was a man of about 50, very heavy built, wearing glasses, and I gained the impression that although he spoke perfect

English, he was a foreigner. After carrying the man clear I looked around for medical assistance and saw an ambulance on the starboard side of the aircraft about 70 yards away. I went across to the ambulance but could find no medical personnel or medical equipment in the ambulance, i.e. stretchers, first aid kits, splints etc. I did notice however that other people on the ground around the aircraft were receiving medical attention and it is possible that the equipment of the ambulance was already being deployed. I returned to the injured man, made him as comfortable as I could and after what appeared to me to be a long time, between five to ten minutes, an ambulance man came over. I explained to him that the injured man had probably a broken leg; after a quick examination he left and returned immediately with a first aid kit, and later obtained a splint. This was applied to the injured man's leg; the bandages in the first aid box were not long enough to strap the splint to the injured man, and the splint was tied on eventually with rags. A doctor and nurse had by this time arrived and supervised the application of the splint, and the injured man was taken away by an ambulance.

Andrew McCarthy remembered that the first medical assistance that was available at the aircraft side came from the BOAC nursing sisters based at Speedbird House, along the southern part of the perimeter road, assisted, at first, by British Eagle employees and some of the BOAC crew managers. The staff magazine *BOAC News* reported the following week that:

Doctors were at the scene within minutes. Dr Ian Dawson left the medical centre opposite Hatton Cross and was quickly joined by Dr J. Graham Taylor, the Director of Medical Services of the joint BOAC-BEA service, and Dr Alan Peffers. The duty medical officer at the central area, Dr Donald McKenzie, was on his way back from London and went straight in.

Dr Peter Richards came from the north side medical unit to join Dr Rory Barnes in preparing the central area medical unit for the first arrivals.

...In the central area unit the duty nursing sisters, Mary Summers, Var Wong, and Hilary Askham were joined by other medical staff and by London Station volunteers [BOAC ground staff at Heathrow] with medical knowledge.

The arrival of fire engines at the aircraft side was slow and the two engines that followed the aircraft down the runway appeared to be poorly equipped and did not manage to keep the fire at bay for very long. Arnold Gosnold noticed:

...two fire engines position themselves to the rear of the aircraft; one at the rear of the tailplane and the other further left. I estimate about half a minute elapsed between the time the aircraft stopped and the fire engines arrived; in any case people were evacuating the aircraft by the time they arrived. As far as I could see one appliance (the rear one) was hosing the port rear part of the aircraft, certainly water or foam from one of the appliances did not even reach the aircraft, it only dribbled out the end of the hose. I then saw other fire engines being led by a C.O.2. tender approach the left front part of the aircraft; there appeared to me to be a very long time between the arrival of the first two fire engines and these latter appliances. The C.O.2. tender started spraying gas from a position approximately 20 yards from the aircraft and it drove into the port wing root still spraying; the fire appeared to be immediately blanketed by the gas. It then appeared to run out of product as did the two engines at the rear of the aircraft and the fire once again took a tremendous hold of the aircraft, and seemed to me to be uncontrollable.

At a later stage, perhaps ten minutes after the accident occurred the London Fire Brigade arrived; whereupon the picture altered, somebody took command and the fire was very soon under control; blanketed in foam.

Meanwhile, in the smoke filled cabin, passengers were still trying to get out as quickly as they could. Sisters Helena and Dorothy Morcom Taylor had not wanted to leave the stricken plane by the over-wing exits, fearing that they would be badly injured if they had to jump onto the ground from such a height.

In any case they had not yet managed to get their camera equipment out of their hand luggage and had no intentions of leaving it behind, despite the fact that their lives were at stake. They recounted later that, as the aircraft landed, music was playing in the cabin and likened it to the passengers fleeing from the sinking *Titanic* as the orchestra played. Having safely gathered their cameras together they were delighted to find that the starboard forward chute was now in place and happily slid down it, with their cameras, to safety.

For those passengers further down the cabin, especially those at the back where the fire was worse, the chance of escape was diminishing. The flames from the port side of the aircraft were rapidly spreading underneath the fuselage and the smoke and fumes were choking them. When the fuel tank exploded the resultant spread of the fire meant that there was no longer a safe side to leave the aircraft; every exit now had its own dangers and it was also becoming difficult to see and to breathe. Richard Hamond said that the smoke was black and greasy and the smell was worse than that of burning rubber.

After eighteen passengers – fourteen men and four women – had made their escape through the over-wing exit, Neville Davis-Gordon stopped any more getting out this way for fear that they would be killed by the fire that was enveloping the wing. Patricia Hay and her daughter Diane were already on the wing when the Chief Steward decided that it was too dangerous to continue using this opening and they had to be helped back into the cabin from where they made their way to the front and slid down the chute at the starboard galley door. The rest of the Hay family also escaped through the front starboard exit.

Although there had been a lot of noise when passengers realized the aircraft was on fire, there was very little panic and most people got out of their seats quickly and into the aisle to shuffle forward towards the only serviceable chute and their escape. Richard Hamond was standing behind a girl of about twelve who was very upset and seemed to him to be on the verge of hysteria. As they made their way forward he kept slapping her on the back and telling her to stop panicking and by the time they reached the door he said she had become much calmer and went down the chute without any further problems. When he reached the ground Dr Hamond bumped into a young man who, he discovered, was flying out to Singapore to join a ship. They chatted as they hurried away from the aircraft and came across a woman in a pretty floral dress who was dazed and obviously suffering from shock. She was being supported by a man of slight build and they were not making good progress away from the fire so Dr Hamond and the young sailor took an arm each and ran with the woman towards the grass where they sat her down. They then saw another similarly dressed woman and rushed her away from the aircraft as well, sitting her down next to the other woman and draping their own coats around the women's shoulders.

At the back of the aircraft Bryan Taylor had opened the exit on the starboard side and had fixed the chute in place. Jane began directing passengers towards it but no one managed to get out through this door before the chute twisted and became unusable. Bryan left Jane to help the passengers, and climbed down the chute himself to straighten it. Once on the ground he was unable to re-enter the aircraft but shepherded people away from the inferno as they reached the ground from all the exits that were in use. When Fred Pragnell put his daughter Dawn onto the chute and pushed her down Bryan Taylor caught her and carried her to safety. She was followed by Vera Pragnell and then Steven. As he went to slide down the chute, the aircraft moved and Steven hit his head and nearly fell over the side. When he reached the bottom Fred, who had made his escape immediately behind his son, scooped him up and ran with him as fast as he could. While he was running Fred turned and heard a fireman yell to him to get away as fast as he could as the aircraft was going to explode. As they got to the edge of the runway there was a huge explosion. Stunned, the family stood looking at the blazing aircraft. Another passenger came up to them and spoke to Fred:

> I think he was Italian; he couldn't speak much English but he came up to me and held up his hand. There were un-popped blisters on his ears, his eyes were red and weeping

from the smoke, as ours were...I gave him my hankie and wished him well.

Inside the cabin Jane had managed to get two men and three women onto the rear chute before sparks and flames from under the fuselage set it on fire and it burst. She continued to direct passengers towards the open doorway as there was a queue of people facing the other way and heading towards the front starboard door where the chute was still intact. She encouraged a couple to jump. Although the risk of being injured was great, their options were so limited that it was worth taking the chance rather than staying onboard and trying to get to a serviceable exit.

Esther Cohen, who had been brought onboard the aircraft in a wheelchair, was sitting towards the back of the aircraft. The nurse who had attended to her at Heathrow had told the crew that she would be fine once in her seat but she, of course, meant during the course of a normal flight. Flight 712 was anything but normal and if Mrs Cohen was to stand a chance of surviving she would need a lot of assistance to get out of the aircraft. Although the nurse had attended to the passenger's medical and personal needs, Esther Cohen could not walk and was unable to do anything for herself. She was also quite a large lady who would have been difficult to move in the confines of a row of aircraft seats.[8]

Andrew McCarthy thinks that Mrs Cohen may have been sitting alongside the Shearers – Annie and Catherine – and that this made it difficult for the two Australians to leave their seats. There may also have been another reason why they were slow in getting up. Brian Cooper, also at the back of the aircraft, saw two women, possibly the Shearers, who seemed to be rigid with fear and who were therefore unable to move at all. All efforts to help them fell on deaf ears as they didn't respond to any pleas for them to save themselves. Eventually Annie Shearer did manage to get out of her seat and left the aircraft by the same route as most of the surviving passengers.

Brian soon realized that he had problems of his own. When he stood up to leave his seat he became separated from his wife, Shirley, and their youngest son, four year old Andrew. He looked for his two other children but since they were sitting in seats two rows forward of him and his wife, Kevin and Jacqueline were being swept along towards the front of the aircraft and away from where they had last seen their parents and brother. Andrew had fallen over when leaving his seat but his mother hadn't seen this and couldn't see where he had gone. The smoke and fumes were getting worse by the second as Shirley frantically searched for her little boy. Brian by this time was at the starboard rear exit where Jane was trying to get passengers to jump thorough the open doorway onto the concrete although there was no safety device to break their falls. Seeing Brian hesitate for a moment, Jane gave him a powerful shove and he fell through the opening onto the runway below. Shirley had discovered to her horror that poor little Andrew was on the floor, being trampled by other passengers trying to get to the exit and, with a huge effort, managed to grab him and throw him out of the same opening that her husband had fallen from, to safety. Miraculously Andrew's only injury was a grazed knee. Shirley then jumped herself, banging her left knee badly as she landed and rolling underneath the fuselage towards the flames.

On the ground Brian was frantically searching for his family. He found Andrew and heard Shirley calling. With the help of a policeman he managed to pull his wife from under the aircraft and help her to a safe place. He then found Kevin who had used the forward chute to leave Whisky Echo. The boy was distraught as he knew that his sister was still on the aircraft but he had been unable to grab her before someone pushed him down the chute. He was shouting that his sister was still onboard and tried to fight his way back so that he could get onto the aircraft again and find Jacqueline but it was impossible. There were still people escaping from the forward door and the rescue workers on the ground were trying to get the survivors away from the burning wreckage as quickly as they could. Neither he nor his father could do anything to help Jacqueline except tell everyone that the little girl was still missing.

The final few moments of the evacuation were a nightmare of smoke and flames. Visibility was virtually nil and it was

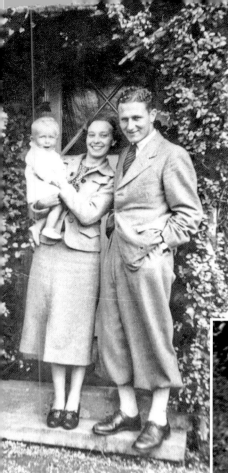

Jane Harrison's parents, Lena and Alan aged approximately twenty-three and twenty-four. Lena Harrison is holding her nephew, Patrick Worthington.
(via Patrick Worthington)

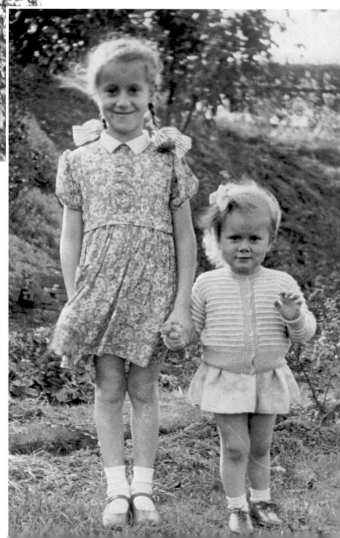

Jane Harrison (right)
with her sister Sue.
(via Sue Buck)

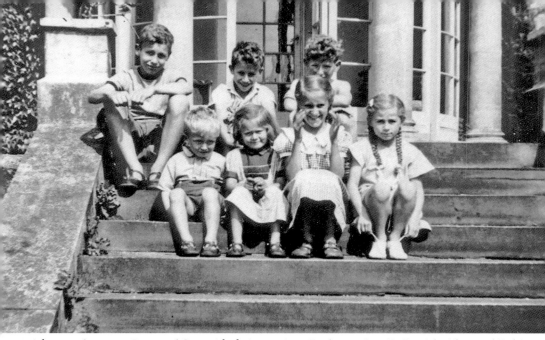

A happy day out – Jane and Sue with their cousins. Back row, L to R: Patrick, Alan and Robin. Front row, L to R: Martin, Jane, Sue and Carol. *(via Patrick Worthington)*

Jane, third from left, was a bridesmaid at the wedding of her school friend Sheila Turton to John Walkington in 1964. *(via Sheila Walkington)*

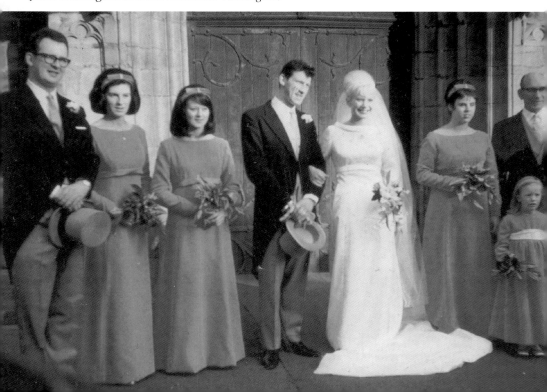

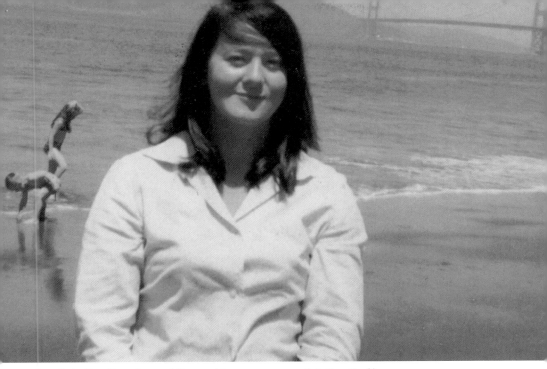

e on a beach in San Francisco while working as a nanny. *(via Sue Buck)*

e with Jeffrey Allende, the little boy she was employed to care for, while in San Francisco.
Sue Buck)

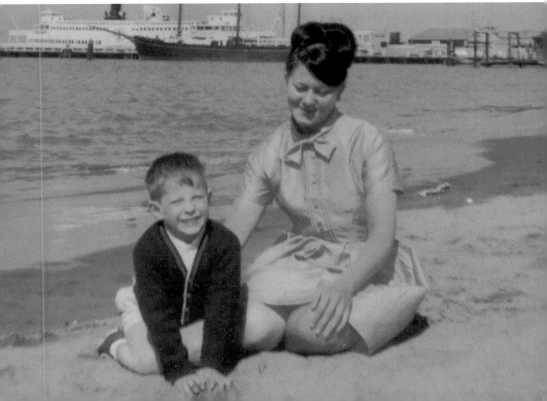

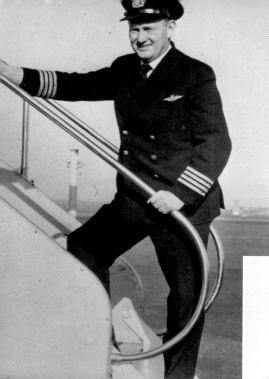

Captain Cliff Taylor, who made a brilliant emergency landing in the burning 707, Whisky Echo, on 8 April 1968. (via Mrs Audrey Taylor)

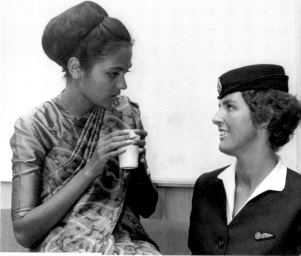

Stewardesses Jennifer Suares and Rosalind Unwin. (via Andrew McCar

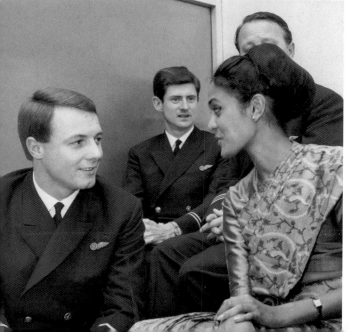

Some more of Whisky Echo's cabin c
L to R: Bryan Taylor, Andrew McCar
and Jennifer Suares. Neville Davis-
Gordon is behind Miss Suares.
(via Andrew McCarthy)

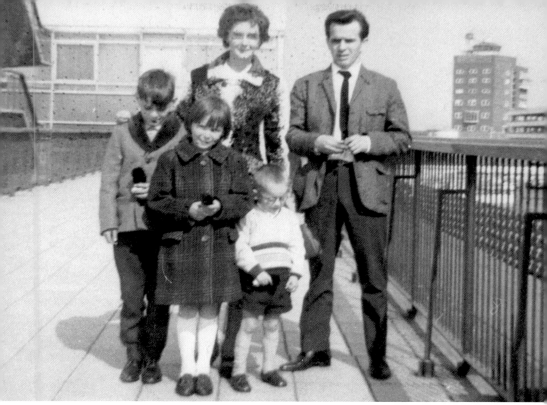

...ey and Brian Cooper with their children (L to R) Kevin, Jacqueline and Andrew at Heathrow airport ...before they boarded Whisky Echo to emigrate to Perth, Australia. *(via Shirley Cooper)*

...ng 707 Whisky Echo in its old livery. The two over-wing exits are beneath the 'O' and 'A' of BOAC. ...rear exit, below and slightly left of the '707' on the fuselage, was where Jane Harrison pushed out ...assengers that she saved. *(© Peter R. Keating via John Wegg)*

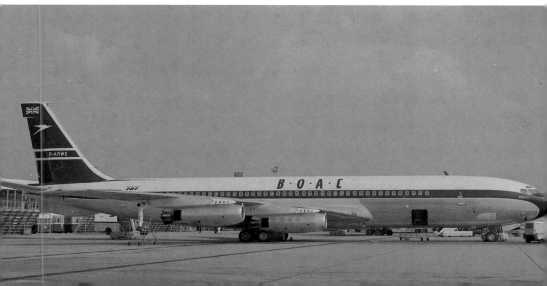

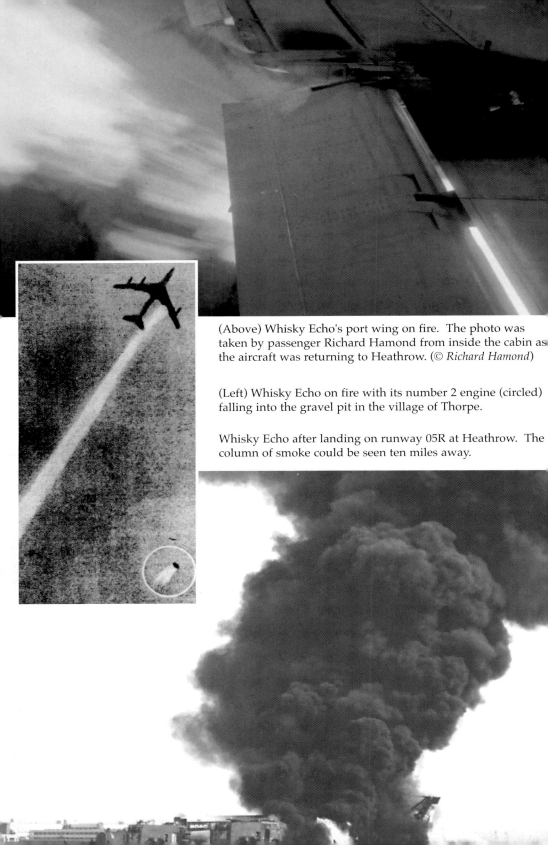

(Above) Whisky Echo's port wing on fire. The photo was taken by passenger Richard Hamond from inside the cabin as the aircraft was returning to Heathrow. (© *Richard Hamond*)

(Left) Whisky Echo on fire with its number 2 engine (circled) falling into the gravel pit in the village of Thorpe.

Whisky Echo after landing on runway 05R at Heathrow. The column of smoke could be seen ten miles away.

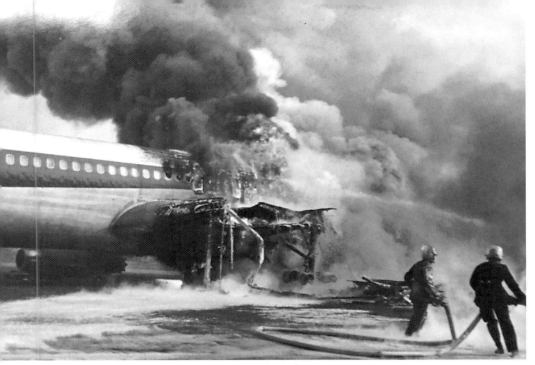

The stub of the port wing of Whisky Echo from which the number 2 engine fell. Two firemen pull a hand line into position to fight the fire.

Police at the scene of the accident. This photo was taken at the moment that an explosion blasted a huge hole in the top of the fuselage and is likely to have been caused by the aircraft's emergency oxygen supply igniting.

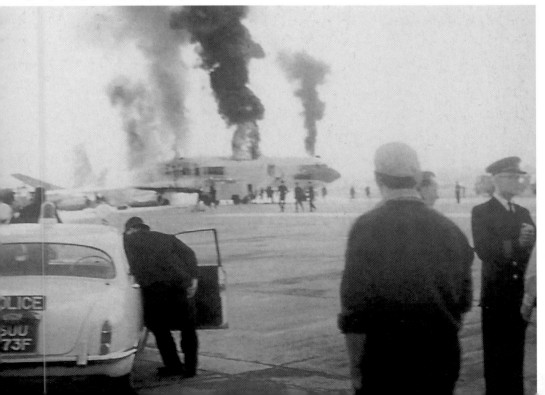

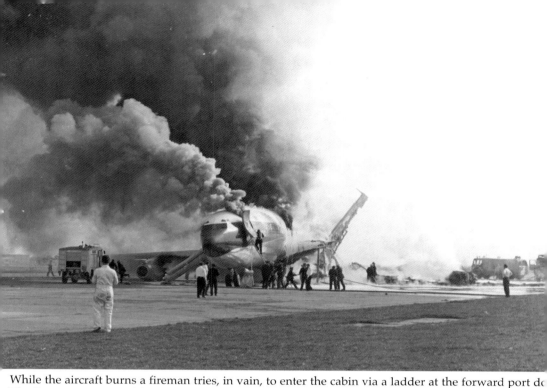

While the aircraft burns a fireman tries, in vain, to enter the cabin via a ladder at the forward port do
The firemen were not able to get onboard until after the fire had been extinguished because they did
not have any protective clothing and the intense heat made it impossible. The chute at the passenger
door is still inflated. *(via John Hutchinson)*

Whisky Echo after the fire had been put out. Note the rope hanging from the cockpit window, which
three of the four pilots used to make their escape, and the now deflated passenger chute down which
most of the survivors escaped.

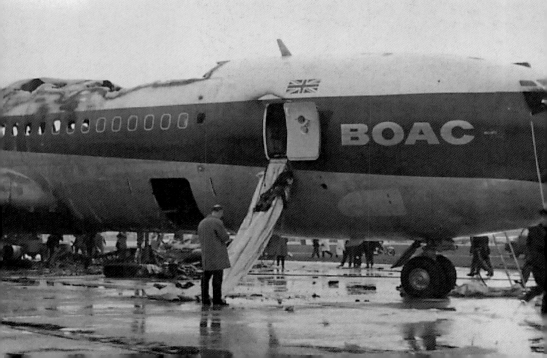

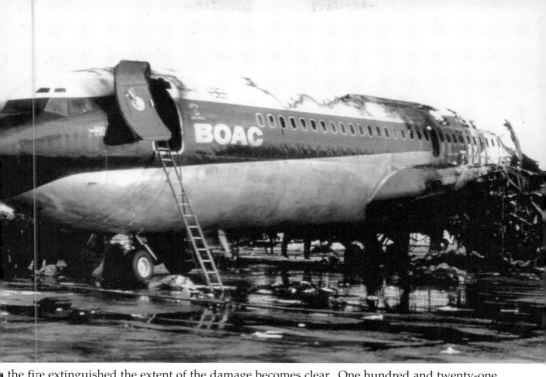

With the fire extinguished the extent of the damage becomes clear. One hundred and twenty-one people escaped from the inferno. (© *Reg Findlay*)

The almost unrecognizable remains of the port wing and undercarriage.

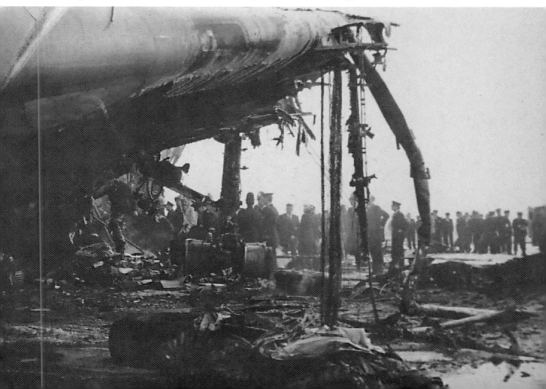

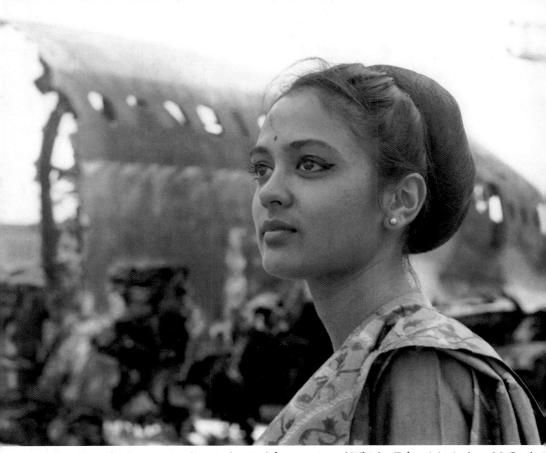

Stewardess Jennifer Suares standing in front of the remains of Whisky Echo. *(via Andrew McCarthy)*

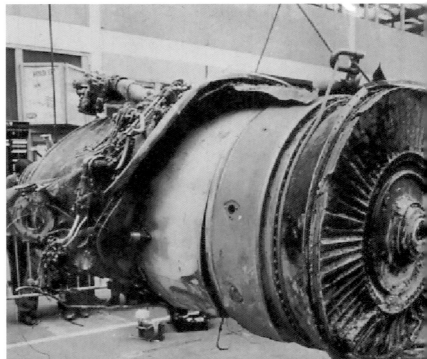

The number 2 engine after recovery from the water filled gravel pit in Thorpe.

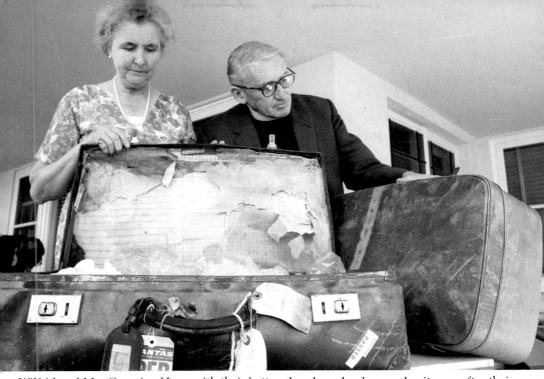

on Wilfrid and Mrs Georgina Henn with their battered and smoke-damaged suitcases after their
val in Perth. *(Reproduced Courtesy West Australian Newspapers)*

viving passenger Eric Blower with his wife Rita and daughter Nicola soon after they settled in
h. *(via Eric Blower)*

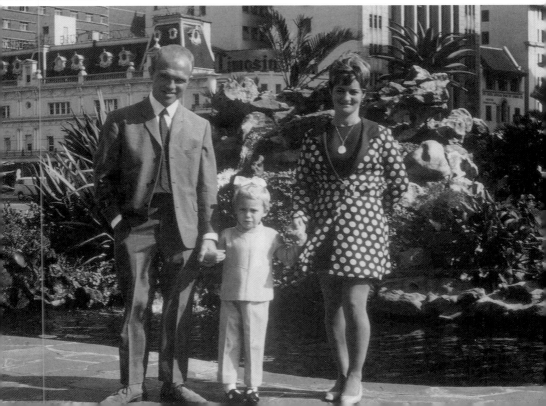

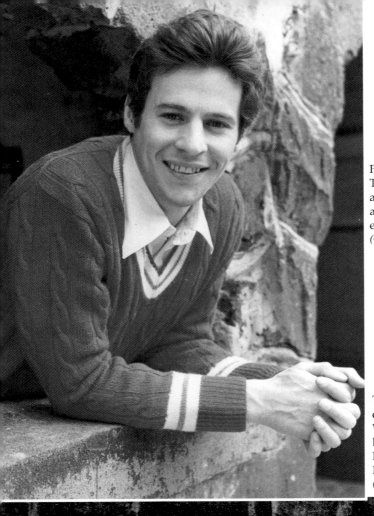

Pop singer Mark Wynter. This photo was taken a week after his wedding in Melbourne and less than a month after his escape from Whisky Echo.
(© Mark Wynter)

The Hay children who were emigrating to Australia from Warsash near Southampton. Back row: Diane and Trevor. Front row, L to R: Lorraine, Kevin and Cheryl.
(via Trevor Hay)

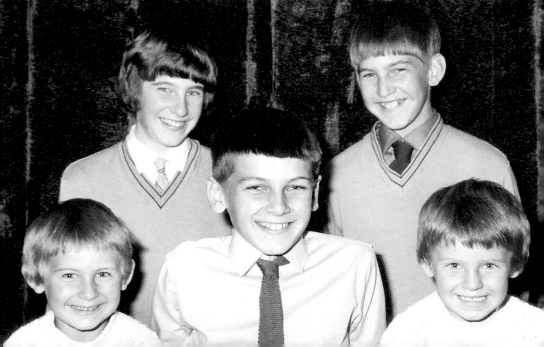

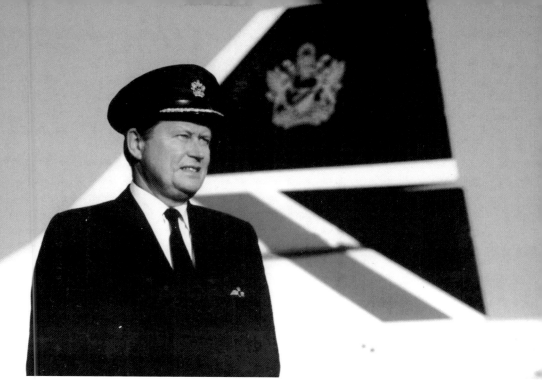

...ain John Hutchinson in front of Concorde, the aircraft he flew for fifteen years. On 8 April 1968 ...was Acting First Officer onboard Whisky Echo. *(via John Hutchinson)*

...wreckage of Whisky Echo after it had been moved to the maintenance area. *(© Reg Findlay)*

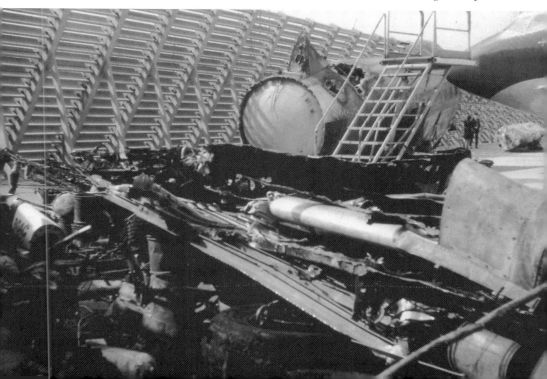

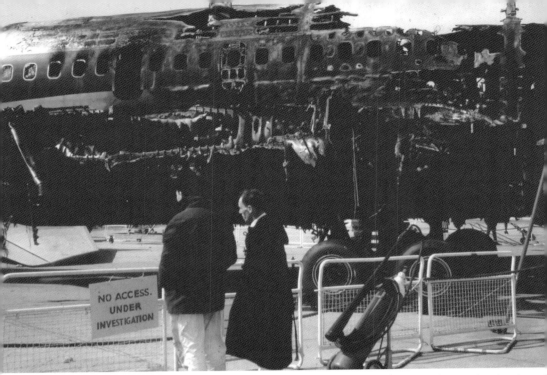

The remains of the aircraft cordoned off in the maintenance area for the official investigation into t
cause of the accident. (© *Reg Findlay*)

TWA Boeing 707 N28714 at Athens airport on 6 June 1973. Four years before, when registered as
N776TW, its cockpit and nose section had been destroyed by a terrorist bomb in Damascus. It was
replaced by the cockpit and nose section from Whisky Echo, the only part of the aircraft to survive
fire. (© *Kjell Nilsson*)

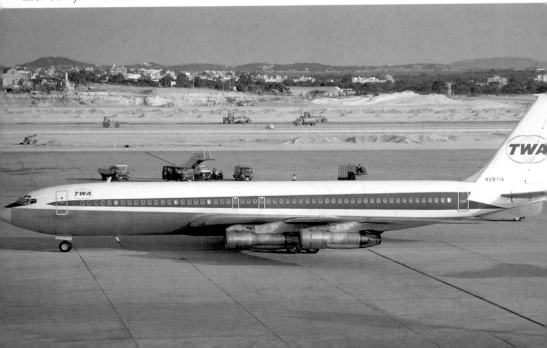

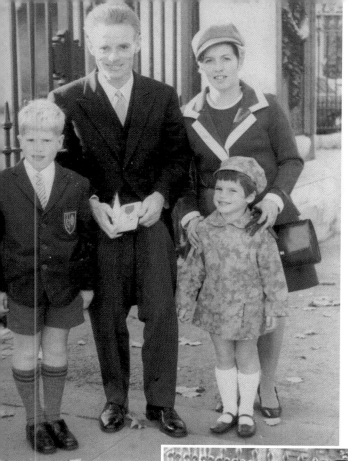

Air Traffic Controller John Davis, with his wife Jaqi and children Andrew and Linda, outside Buckingham Palace following the award of his MBE. *(via John Davis)*

Chief Steward Neville Davis-Gordon holding the British Empire Medal for Gallantry that he was given following the accident. He was accompanied to the Palace for the investiture by his wife Diddy and daughter Carole. *(via Diddy Davis-Gordon)*

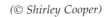
(© Shirley Cooper)

Jacqueline Cooper
12 December 1959 – 8 April 1968

Jane Harrison, GC
24 May 1945 – 8 April 1968

(via Sue Buck)

becoming almost impossible to breathe. When the cabin crew were as sure as they could be that there was no one else left on board they began their own escape. Bryan Taylor had, of course, already left and Neville Davis-Gordon, Jennifer Suares, Rosalind Unwin and Andrew McCarthy all left via the starboard galley door. Rosalind commented that they would have had to leave then anyway as the cabin floor was sagging and she felt that had they stayed a moment longer it would have collapsed completely, sending them to their deaths in the blazing cargo compartments below. There had already been a series of explosions and, with the fire still raging, the chances of avoiding any more, when the aircraft still contained most of its fuel load, were very slight. The remainder of the cockpit crew also made their escape at this point. Thomas Hicks had already left the aircraft in order to straighten the forward port chute and Geoff Moss, the check captain, went down the chute on the starboard side in a very brief gap between passengers. Francis Kirkland left via the rope hanging from the sliding cockpit window.

John Hutchinson and Cliff Taylor stood at the front of the cabin, shouting to check that everyone had left the aircraft. They could hardly see their hands in front of their faces at this point and were finding it difficult to breathe. Hearing no replies to their calls, they went back into the cockpit to escape through the window. Cliff Taylor then used the rope to reach the ground and finally so too did John Hutchinson. As he climbed out of the window and hung onto the sill for a brief moment, a ring that he was wearing caught in the rope and nearly broke his finger. A fireman on the ground shouted at him to let go and come down the rope, not knowing the reason for his hesitation and although he tried to control his descent, his hands were so hot and sweaty that the rope slithered through them and he found himself sliding uncontrollably to the ground. The rope used for this escape route was made of nylon and he suffered rope burns while getting off the aircraft. He still wears the ring that caught in the rope and it has a dent in it to this day.

BEA engineer John Webb was still at the aircraft side and:

... helped to carry a lady away, who was in a state of shock and later during the evacuation after the fire had worsened and there had been a number of explosions I helped to drag a young man, apparently unconscious, laying by the chute. I believe he must have been one of the last to evacuate the aircraft, his face and clothing were black and he was in an apparent choked and shocked condition. He was taken by an ambulance to safety. Soon after the young man left I noticed a crew member coming down the rope from the starboard cockpit window and I think that this was the termination of the evacuation.

Despite the unanswered calls made through the cabin there were still passengers who had not yet managed to escape. As she was about to leave, Jane either heard someone calling to her or perhaps realized that there were people on the ground still waiting for their loved ones to emerge from the wreckage. The aircraft was burning out of control, the air was thick with smoke and fumes and Jane was standing in the worst affected part of it. The aircraft's back had been broken and her only escape route would have been to jump through the door where she had pushed Brian Cooper. Bryan Taylor had last seen her when he reached the ground himself although she disappeared from view soon afterwards. Stewardess Jennifer Suares remembered that the last time she had seen Jane was soon after Whisky Echo landed when she looked towards the rear of the aircraft, before the smoke became too thick to see anything, and saw Jane standing in the aisle about six rows from the back. On the ground several passengers recalled seeing her in the doorway, about to leave the aircraft, and then she turned and went back into the cabin. She obviously knew what the rest of the crew and ground staff did not at that time, that widowed Mary Smith, who had been going to Australia to visit her brothers, was still there; so was Esther Cohen, who was returning to her home in Haifa and who couldn't walk. The young Australian teacher Catherine Shearer, who had either been trapped in her seat and unable to climb over Mrs Cohen or had succumbed to her fear and been unable to move, was still onboard. Blonde haired little Jacqueline Cooper, who Kevin, her brother, had tried so hard to save, was still there too. Jane couldn't leave them to their fate and so, with no thought for her own safety, although she must have known that she had very little chance of survival, went back into the inferno and was never seen alive again.

Chapter 6

The Evening News

As the last crew members left the aircraft and assembled on the runway Neville Gordon-Davis:

> ...took a head count of my cabin crew and found that Miss Harrison was missing. I went back to the aircraft and told one of the firemen that one of my girls was still in there, and he said he would do what he could but I could see that the whole of the tail area was a blazing inferno. I waited around tending to the injured and helped putting them into the ambulance. It was after that, that with the other four of my crew I left in the Police van for the Medical section.

As each of the cabin crew came down the chute and landed on the runway, they looked around them to satisfy themselves that their colleagues were safe. Rosalind Unwin remembers that when she made her escape she was followed by Andrew McCarthy and then Neville Davis-Gordon. Jennifer Suares was there and Rosalind spotted Bryan Taylor but she could not see Jane. She asked Bryan if he knew where she was:

> He did not know – I believed the worst as we were told that she had probably been taken to hospital. I knew better. Instinct? I don't think that Bryan or I believed she was alive.

At the bottom of the chute Rosalind saw someone she did know – an employee of British Eagle also called Brian who she had once dated. He went back to his office and telephoned Rosalind's mother to tell her that he had seen Rosalind and that she was quite safe.

When they all reached the medical centre the cabin crew were examined by Dr Atholl Hepburn. The cockpit crew, who had walked to the centre, were seen by Dr Alan Sibbald, an extremely popular member of the BOAC medical team and described by John Hutchinson as 'a fantastic chap'. The cabin crew again asked about Jane and were again told that she had probably gone to hospital. By now none of them believed it. One by one they were all examined and released to go home. The cockpit crew were told that they had to be back at the airport the following morning when the airline's own enquiry into what had gone wrong would begin.

Andrew McCarthy lived close to the airport and having been given the clearance from the doctor went home to his wife Christina and his young daughter.

Rosalind Unwin was very grateful to her British Eagle friend for telephoning her mother as she discovered later that the first broadcast that her family had heard had said that 100 people were feared dead in the accident. Because of that phone call the entire family knew she was safe, as Mrs Unwin contacted everyone with the good news. Rosalind herself was checked by the doctor at the medical centre and, apart from a slight burn on the inside of her left arm, was passed as fit. She was still filthy from the smoke but was anxious to get home. Her bag containing her car keys had been destroyed in the fire so she telephoned her boyfriend, Peter Edgar, and asked him to go to her parents' house and get the spare set and a saw to remove the crook lock and then come and get her. This was a lengthy trip for Peter and he eventually arrived at Heathrow at about 8:30 – 9:00 p.m. He brought with him his sister and her boyfriend who drove his car home while he drove Rosalind's. Although they arrived back in Coventry very late that evening Rosalind found a group of photographers waiting for her at her parents' front gate. She, along with the other crew members, had been briefed before leaving Heathrow not to speak to the press until more was known about the accident and they had been given the go-ahead from BOAC. She pushed silently past the photographers, helped by Peter, who then left her in the care of her parents.

At her home in Hertfordshire, John Hutchinson's wife Sue had been making the most of the fine weather to do some gardening. Her two sons were inside the house watching *Blue Peter* on the television when suddenly there was a break in the programme to announce that there had been a serious accident at Heathrow. The boys listened to what was being said about a BOAC aircraft bound for Australia catching fire and then one of them ran out into the garden to tell his mother that, 'Dad's plane is on fire'. Sue reassured her son that it couldn't be the same aircraft as John had left home that morning and should have been well on his way to Australia by then. However, she was then confronted by her neighbour who had chatted to John that morning and who said that the flight number that was being given on the television was the same one that John had told her he was taking. Then the phone rang. When Sue answered it she found it was from someone at BOAC asking if her husband was at home. Puzzled, and by now beginning to worry, she answered that he was taking a flight out to Australia that day and was not at home. The caller thanked her and hung up. This really worried her but then the phone rang again and she was relieved to find that it was John. He told her that there had been an accident at Heathrow and that because of it his flight to Australia had been cancelled and that he would be coming home that evening. He didn't mention the ordeal he had just been through and Sue remembers thinking that now he would be able to spend some time with the children during their Easter holidays. She cleared up her gardening tools and went back indoors to do some ironing while waiting for John to come home.

The phone rang once more. It was another call from BOAC but this time it was someone telling her about the accident and breaking the news that they were very sorry to have to tell her but her husband had been on board the aircraft that had caught fire and could not be accounted for. Sue was now really confused and said that he was fine – she had just spoken to him! The caller was also confused and wanted to know where he had called from. Eventually Sue received another call, this time from Dr Sibbald, to tell her that John was indeed safe and that he would be bringing him home a little later. It was never really explained satisfactorily how the muddle had occurred.

Doctor Sibbald had asked John where he lived and when he told him, said that he, too, lived in Hertfordshire and would give him a lift on his way home. It was only when they were on the way to John's house that he discovered that the doctor lived miles away in the completely opposite direction. As they approached John's home Dr Sibbald asked him the name of his local pub. John told him it was the Jolly Waggoner and directed the doctor to it. He was still wearing his uniform, filthy and smelling of the smoke from the fire and, from the telltale sooty marks on his face and hands and in his hair, it was obvious that he had been through a terrible ordeal. Oblivious to the stares of the other customers, Dr Sibbald took him into the pub and bought him two large whiskies. When he had finished his drinks the doctor then took him home and gave Sue some tablets to give to him, telling her that he was still in shock. Having been a nurse herself she knew how to take care of him and Doctor Sibbald left John in his wife's capable hands and set off on the long journey back to his own home.

Apart from the emergency services and airline staff, the first people to rush to the scene of the fire were BOAC chairman, Sir Giles Guthrie, accompanied by deputy chairman, Keith Granville, and Secretary of State at the Board of Trade, John Mallalieu. The scene, as the photos show, was one of utter devastation. The aircraft was almost totally destroyed; the only part that remained intact was the cockpit. On the ground were the charred remains – wheels with their tyres burnt away; blobs of aluminium where the aircraft had become so hot that its skin had melted; the port wing detached from the fuselage and the remaining engine from that wing, broken and burnt on the concrete; the wreckage of the battered structure looking like the skeleton of an enormous whale that had, long ago, left the safety of the sea and died on the beach where it had been stranded, its bones stripped of flesh. At the front, a deflated escape chute hung limply from the doorway through which so many people had escaped; from the cockpit window dangled the rope down which three of the four pilots had clambered to safety. On the ground around the wreckage were the remains of the aircraft's cargo and mail; charred and tangled boxes and sacks, resting forlornly in pools of water, foam and fuel. More poignantly were the personal belongings of the passengers – the twisted frame of a child's pushchair; the blackened remains of a teddy bear; suitcases; books; passports. The sight that greeted Sir Giles was of firemen and police sifting through the wreckage, pulling out anything that they thought might be salvaged. These items were taken to the Airport Police Headquarters gymnasium where they were painstakingly catalogued.

One of the more urgent tasks after the fire had been extinguished was to locate the radioactive package that had been part of the aircraft's cargo. At 16:45 the occupational health engineer from the Air Corporations Joint Medical Service, Mr D. Doran, arrived at the crash scene. In a report made the following day he described how the package was finally located and how its mishandling by the emergency services could have resulted in yet more tragedy:

> I learnt that a radioactive cargo consignment was aboard the aircraft. Responsibility for detection and retrieval rests with the B.A.A. Airport Fire Service and a fire officer with a radiation monitor was in fact on site.
>
> Eventually I was shown a partly burned package which was thought to be the radioactive consignment and had been isolated. The type of packaging was similar to that used for some types of beta-emitting radioisotope. I was informed that "Amersham"[1] had already monitored it and cleared it for disposal by BOAC: my informant added that a low (and safe) radiation dose-rate figure had been quoted.
>
> As such clearance by Amersham seemed most unlikely I asked the fire officer with the monitor to recheck. He obtained no reading – which suggested either that the package was not a beta-emitting radioactive consignment or that his instrument was faulty. I then obtained a more sensitive type of monitor from my own office, returned to the site and confirmed that this package was not the radioactive consignment.
>
> Subsequently I received a message that what appeared to be a radioactive consignment was lying in the Airport Police Headquarters gymnasium where all salvaged cargo, etc. was

being assembled. Almost simultaneously I learnt that two Amersham officials had arrived at London Station Duty Room.

I collected these officials (Mr. G. Dancer, Mr. W. Chiswell) from the Duty Room and we went together to the Police gymnasium. The consignment had lost its outer packaging but the main container, though dented and scorched was proved, by monitoring, to be intact. Therefore there was no risk of contamination spread.

I was informed by the Police that as this item had not yet been listed it could be taken away without formality. I took the opportunity to ask the BOAC Head Loader who apparently had loaded the aircraft whether there had been more than one radioactive consignment; he confirmed my earlier information that there had only been one.

...I assured those present who had handled the consignment that the dose-rate was such that anyone handling it for short periods would be subjected to no health hazard whatever. Left in the Police gymnasium, however, it would have represented a potential hazard.

When news of the accident was received at BOAC's London terminal an incident room was set up and staff were called in to man the phones and answer calls from worried family and friends of those who had been on board Whisky Echo. As they received each new scrap of news, details were written on boards around the room so that the airline could ensure that each passenger could be accounted for. The task itself proved to be more difficult than one would suppose. The passengers who had escaped without injury and had congregated at the British Eagle buildings or had simply sat down on the grass bordering the runway were put in BOAC buses and taken to the British Airport Authority's Alcock and Brown VIP suite. Here they were given food and drink and the chance to relax while BOAC arranged hotel accommodation for the night. Their details were easy to record but the problem that made it impossible to get an exact count of the fatalities until very late that night was that some passengers had simply run from the blazing aircraft and had kept running right off the airport, into the surrounding streets, and had then made their way home without informing anyone from the airline what they were doing. In the days before the strict security that is now in place at all airports, it was quite easy to leave the customs and immigration area – what is known as 'airside' – without being stopped by anyone. In their shocked state, these passengers just wanted to get to the comfort of their own homes as fast as possible and it didn't occur to any one of them that they might have been presumed dead. The BOAC staff at the incident room had to go through the passenger list and find the contact details of those who were missing. Telephone numbers and addresses were given to the police who followed up these leads and eventually, at around 23:00, were able to account for everyone who had been on board. In a telegram, sent by R.H. Morgan at Boeing to all Boeing Commercial Field Service bases, giving details of the accident, the number of dead had been correctly identified including the fact that there were four passengers and one crew member. That telegram was timed at 3:05 PST[2] which confirmed the time that everyone was eventually accounted for.

Two local hospitals, Ashford and Hillingdon, had taken injured passengers into their care and the names of these passengers were also easy to obtain. One of them was singer Mark Wynter. After he jumped off the starboard wing and onto the runway he had escaped to the British Eagle offices. Having had a drink and a rest he felt a little better and tried to stand up but found that he couldn't. Although he had been able to run away from the blazing aircraft and had helped another passenger to escape as well, it had been his survival instinct that had allowed him to get clear of the aircraft, for when he jumped he had actually injured himself, something he had not realized until he tried to stand. He was taken to Hillingdon hospital from where he called both his mother and his agent to let them know he was safe. When doctors examined him they found that he had sprained his left ankle and broken a bone in his right foot. Mark's agent, Ian Bevan, who lived in Mayfair, arranged for him to be transferred to St George's Hospital at Hyde Park Corner where his right leg was put in plaster up to the knee and when he was discharged he went to Mr Bevan's flat to recover.

Katriel Katz was also taken to Hillingdon hospital where he, along with other passengers from Whisky Echo, was visited by steward Andrew McCarthy the next day. Andrew was shocked by the Israeli's condition and was concerned that perhaps the accident would claim one more victim as Mr Katz seemed to him to be in a very bad state. He, however, was made of sterner stuff than most people believed and, after a few days began to improve. He eventually made a good recovery and died, twenty years later, at the age of eighty.

Retired teacher Nellie Abbott was another of the passengers taken to Hillingdon hospital. While the aircraft had been making its desperate return to Heathrow, she had filmed the fire and, when she left the aircraft, had managed to take her cine camera with her. Still photos were made from parts of her film and she herself was photographed in her hospital bed the following day holding in one hand a copy of the *Daily Mirror* newspaper, with the account of the accident, and, curiously, in her other hand a lighted cigarette; government health warnings and hospital regulations being more lax in those days than they are today! These photographs appeared in an article in the French magazine, *Paris Match*.

The photo that Frank Tyler had taken from the top of the Queen's Building was highly sought after in the hours following the accident. Frank recalled that:

I went into work that evening and was persuaded to take the film up to Fleet Street in London, which was then the centre of the newspaper industry. Two of us were given the time off work and we drove up to London and saw a photo editor of UPI – United Press Intl. He offered me £50 for the use of it or a percentage of whatever they sold it for. Little did I know it would end up on the front cover of *Paris Match*; perhaps I should have taken the percentage! That edition contained some b&w pictures taken by passengers on board as well as one of the aircraft coming over the village to the south of the airfield.

I still get a shiver when I think about that afternoon. It seemed a very unreal situation, almost like watching a film.

Young Steven Pragnell, suffering from concussion after hitting his head, had been admitted to Ashford Hospital where he was kept under observation until the following day, while Shirley Cooper was admitted to Hillingdon hospital where her injured left knee was treated. The young mother was photographed at the hospital the day after the accident. Still traumatized by her ordeal she sat, her knee heavily bandaged, clutching her youngest child, Andrew, on her lap, her despair at having lost her only daughter clearly visible on her face.

While waiting in the airport's VIP lounge, Eric Blower met another passenger who, he discovered, had been sitting directly behind him on the aircraft:

> He said he had written down all the events on a notepad. He meticulously calculated the advancing rate of the fire by counting the rivets in the wing and, using a stopwatch, timed the rate at which they were being consumed by the fire. In his own words he said that he was a scientist and had written it all down so that if he had died maybe his information would have been salvaged and help in the inquiry.

At first the phones in the Alcock and Brown suite were not working due, the passengers were told, to a complete overload of the airport switchboard and so it was some time before they were able to make calls to their families to let them know they were safe.

Eric Blower described this time as being:

> ...the worst part for me.
> When the phone lines became available we were all allowed to make calls from the many phones around the place. It was a difficult job because the lines were still overloaded and we just had to keep trying. I did eventually get through to my wife's number but she was unable to speak to me; I spoke to her brother.
> My wife had been watching TV at home in Leeds when the programme was interrupted by a news flash showing a burning aircraft on the tarmac at Heathrow. The message describing an Australian bound BOAC 707 aircraft, crash

lands shortly after take off from Heathrow 'with no expected survivors'. When I discovered this it was then I broke down. It was much later in the evening before I was able to speak to Rita.

I stayed at a Heathrow hotel that night and travelled (by train) to Leeds the next day.

Eric was so angry about the television report giving these details before the true facts were known and, in doing so, worrying his wife so badly that felt he would really have liked to sue the BBC.

A news crew from the rival channel, ITV, arrived at Heathrow to film the still smouldering aircraft and, if possible, interview passengers and members of the crew. Richard Hamond decided to push himself forward to be interviewed and gave an account of what had happened during the short flight and the even shorter time it took to evacuate the aircraft. Later that evening, resting on his bed in the Skyways hotel at Heathrow, he was pleased to see the interview on television as it saved him having to contact his family and friends to let them know he was safe.

Air traffic controller, John Davis, also wanted to speak to his family and, when he telephoned his wife, Jaqi, told her that there had been an incident at Heathrow and that he would probably be late getting home. Having finished his cup of tea and written up his notes of what had happened he then had to start again and fill in official reports for the enquiry into the accident, that would soon be held. When he did eventually arrive home that evening Jaqi says he looked absolutely shattered.

In Australia Basil Henn was waiting for news of his parents, Wilfrid and Georgina Henn. Having heard about the fire he had tried to find out what had happened to them but the local BOAC office told him that they had no news. Terrified that they might not have survived, their only son sat on the floor of his living room staring at the phone and praying that they had escaped. He spent an entire day without news and then, eventually, someone from BOAC called to say that they were safe. Despite their ordeal they decided to return to Australia by air, as Mrs Henn was a bad sailor, and so boarded the very next flight bound for Perth. When they arrived they were interviewed and photographed for the *West Australian* newspaper. The photo, which appeared in the edition on 12 April, showed them with their damaged suitcases. It was also reported that they had managed to save a soot blackened bottle of duty free brandy.

At their homes in Yorkshire, Jane Harrison's sister and her friends had watched the news bulletins about the accident on the television.

Sue Buck had seen the evening news report which had said that the crew had all survived and was relieved. Not knowing whether or not her sister had even been onboard the flight, Sue was, however, satisfied that she was safe and well. She had just started to get dinner ready for herself and her husband at their home in Heslington Road, York, when someone knocked on the door. Sue answered it and a man, who looked vaguely familiar to her, asked to speak to Vic, her husband. She called Vic who talked to the man while she went back to the kitchen to get on with the cooking. As she made dinner she was trying to remember where she had seen the man before and, since he had asked for her husband, was worried about what he might want. It never occurred to her that he might have some news about the accident at Heathrow. A moment or so later she heard the front door shut and Vic came into the kitchen to give Sue the devastating news that Jane *had* been onboard the aircraft and that she had died in the fire.

Alan Harrison had been contacted by BOAC at his home in Pinner, Middlesex, and had been told the news about his daughter. Not wanting Sue to find out from the radio or television, and not able to contact her himself because she didn't have a telephone, he had called a friend who lived close to Sue and asked him to go and break the news to his daughter and son-in-law. Sue's first thought was, 'oh, my poor father' because, within the space of little more than ten years he had lost his wife, his second marriage had failed and he had now lost his younger daughter. In her shocked state, Sue pushed her own grief to the back of her mind and concentrated on the practical things that had to be done.

Early the next morning she contacted a friend with whom she

worked and asked her to tell the boss that she wouldn't be coming in that day. Then she went to the station in York to make the long train journey to London to go to Jane's flat. When she arrived she found that Jane's flatmates had already been packing Jane's things for her to take back to Yorkshire, and she fetched Jane's car from the staff car park at Heathrow and drove it and Jane's belongings back home to Yorkshire.

Kay Golightly had a date that Monday evening to go to the cinema with her fiancé. As she got ready she was avidly listening to the news and she, too, was relieved to hear that all members of the crew were safe. Like Sue she wasn't sure that Jane would have been on that flight anyway but the fact that the crew was safe set her mind at rest and she went off to the cinema without a care about her friend.

Having had a late night at the cinema the evening before, Kay had been in a rush to get to work on Tuesday morning and had not had a chance to listen to the news or read a newspaper. She often met her friends at lunchtime in the Wimpy bar that was beneath her office and went down to meet them that day. She couldn't understand why they looked so miserable and asked what was wrong. One of them wanted to know if she had seen the newspaper and, when she said that she hadn't, produced a copy for her to read the main story of the day. Kay was distraught to learn that her friend had been on the aircraft and that, contrary to the first reports, she had died. Devastated by the news she was unable to return to work and was taken home.

Jane's friend, Sheila Turton, by then Sheila Walkington, remembered how she found out about her friend's death:

We saw it on the news and I just knew it was her even before they gave out a name at the next bulletin. I actually received a letter from Jane after that. She must have posted it before she went to work. Jane was 'seeing' a Qantas pilot and was going to tell me all about it when she got back. By then I had a 3 month old daughter as well as my 2½ year old son and I remember being physically sick that day and having to cancel a driving lesson.

In Rome Jane's friend, Margaret Jessop, had heard about the crash and was worried about her:

> The next day I received a post card from her, telling me her news, so thought, thank goodness it's not Jane, then never thought any more about it. Probably there was not much about it in the Italian press, and in any case I couldn't speak Italian, so it was such a shock when I received the press cuttings from my sister with the news that Jane had in fact died. I had nightmares about it for years afterwards.

Patrick Worthington heard the news of the accident at his home in Switzerland. He telephoned the BOAC office in Geneva to ask about his cousin, Jane Harrison. The person he spoke to was pleased to tell him that there was no one of that name on the aircraft but that, coincidentally, the name of the stewardess who had died was Harrison but that her first name was not Jane but Barbara. Patrick immediately knew it had to be Jane and made a call to his family back in England to confirm it. Soon afterwards he wrote a letter to his uncle, Jane's father, expressing affection and admiration for his cousin from himself and his wife:

> If you'd have asked Monique and me a few weeks ago what was the outstanding quality of Jane, Monique would have replied 'courage' and I would have said 'guts'. This is not being wise after the event, Uncle Alan, it was and is our honest opinion formed after her three month stay here in the canton of Neuchatel.

Some of Jane's other friends had also heard that the stewardess was called Barbara Harrison and were comforted, believing that Jane was safe, until they remembered that she never used her actual first name...

***

At Heathrow the emergency workers and those airline staff drafted in to look after passengers from the wrecked aircraft, and trace those who were still missing, worked hard for the rest of the afternoon, throughout the evening and into the early hours of the next day knowing that the repercussions of the flight that had lasted for only three and a half minutes would be felt for many months, even years, to come.

When the blaze onboard Whisky Echo had been contained and it was safe to do so, a fireman clambered into the main part of the wreckage – the almost unrecognizable cabin area – and, close to the rear door, huddled together in the debris that had once been a sleek, shiny jet aircraft, were the bodies of the four women and the little girl who had died.

Chapter 7

Headlines

Following his inspection of the scene of the accident Sir Giles Guthrie was interviewed by reporters. The shaken BOAC chairman issued a statement[1] in which he said:

It is a matter of great credit to everyone concerned that there have been so many survivors.

This was the plane's first flight out – except for a test flight – following a major overhaul.

I shall be conducting my own investigation, apart from that of the Board of Trade. I shall be trying to find out why the fire extinguishers were not working, why the fire warning system was not working, and why the engine caught fire.

The next day the huge task of clearing up the wreckage of the aircraft and the investigations into the reason for the tragedy got underway.

Sir Giles Guthrie's first priority was to send a personal, handwritten message to Jane Harrison's father, Alan. In it he said:

It is with a heavy heart I write to offer you my deep sympathy in the tragic loss of your daughter, Barbara, in our 707 accident yesterday. A complete report is not available yet but it would appear that she died trying to save the lives of others. May I add that you are very much in the thoughts of all of us in BOAC, for we believe Barbara was happy in our airline and we know she made many friends here. She will be sadly missed.

While Sir Giles was writing his letter to Alan Harrison, the Queen's Private Secretary, Lieutenant Colonel Sir Michael Adeane, was sending one to the BOAC chairman in which he said:

> The Queen and The Duke of Edinburgh were so relieved that a major disaster was averted at Heathrow yesterday. Clearly this was due to the skill and coolness of the pilot and I should be grateful if you would express to Captain Taylor the admiration of Her Majesty and His Royal Highness for an outstanding achievement.

Sir Giles replied:

> It will give me much pleasure to make known to Captain Taylor the expression of admiration of Her Majesty and His Royal Highness.

When the cockpit crew had eventually returned to their homes on the evening of 8 April they did so in the knowledge that they would have to return to Heathrow the following day for the enquiries to begin and for the press conference that BOAC had organized. John Hutchinson remembers being embarrassed when he arrived at Heathrow, wearing a red polo necked sweater, and found many of the BOAC staff wearing black ties as a mark of respect to Jane Harrison and the passengers who had died. Because the cockpit and cabin crews had been separated after their escape from the aircraft, John had no idea that anyone had died in the accident until he returned to the airport the following day.

The newspapers on Tuesday 9 April were full of the story of the last flight of Whisky Echo. All other news was relegated to inside pages while the front pages carried dramatic photos of the crippled aircraft and heart rending stories from some of the survivors. The *Daily Express* headline was '121 Alive!' while the *Daily Mirror* led with 'THE MIRACLE From this fiery hell, 121 people got out alive'. *The Guardian*'s headline was a slightly more subdued, but inaccurate, '121 scramble from burning

Boeing after crash landing'. After Cliff Taylor's perfect landing it was an insult to describe it as a 'crash'.

The evening papers were not to be outdone either. Since the accident had occurred in the late afternoon of 8 April the story was too late for that day but, on 9 April, they had the benefit of being able to quote from the press conference held that afternoon. The *Evening Standard* had a photo of Cliff Taylor with his dog, Dinah, under the legend 'Pilot of the blazing Boeing tells what happened in the mid-air drama... "The cookie crumbled in our favour!" ' The front page of *The Evening News* was devoted almost entirely to the story, with photos of the burnt out wreckage of Whisky Echo, stewardess Rosalind Unwin, the entire cockpit crew – Captain Cliff Taylor, with his dog, Dinah, incorrectly identified as 'Blackie', pilots Geoff Moss, Francis Kirkland, John Hutchinson and engineer Thomas Hicks – and Mark Wynter's fiancée, Janeece Corlass, under the headline 'THE CRASH, BY THE PILOT'. The article quoted Captain Taylor as having said:

> Bringing this plane down was a team job. There were five [*sic*] other people on the flight deck and I just happened to be in command.
>
> I have nothing dramatic to tell. We simply went through all those procedures necessary in just such an emergency.
>
> There was no sudden panic. Everyone kept cool and did all that was required of them to the best of their ability.
>
> That is what averted a disaster – the efficiency of my colleagues and the calmness of the passengers.
>
> All praise in the world is due to the cabin staff. The crew were superb. Great men to be associated with. I am proud of them.
>
> My role was to bring the plane down safely. In that I was lucky. Everything was in my favour. The weather conditions were perfect and everything was done to assist me by the air control staff at London Airport.
>
> The others had the job of organising the evacuation of the passengers from the aircraft. That was the most difficult job of all and where the other members of the crew were at their best.

It is to them, for the way in which they did this, that the real praise should go.

Cliff Taylor had also spoken very briefly about Jane during the press conference, when, close to tears, he said:

The cabin staff were superb. One girl sacrificed her life. What more can I say than that? My colleagues were wonderful in clearing the approach. The control tower was magnificent.

In Melbourne, Australia – Janeece Corlass's home town – the story was splashed across the front page of *The Herald* newspaper, with the headline 'JET PILOT SAVES 121 – Grandfather brings in a blazing 707'. Further down the page was a photo of Mark Wynter and an article entitled 'Mark vows to be at the church on time'.

The story of Whisky Echo continued to dominate the national and local press for some days. On Wednesday 10 April, *The Daily Telegraph* featured a story telling how Royal Navy divers had found the missing No. 2 engine. Alongside the article was a photo of Mrs Coretta King in Atlanta, Georgia, at the funeral of her husband, assassinated American civil rights leader, Martin Luther King. Although Dr King had been murdered on 4 April and the reports had been headline news up until 8 April, the tragedy of Whisky Echo relegated even that story to the inside pages of many newspapers until the day of his funeral.

While the nation was learning every detail it could about the accident, many different arrangements were being made as a result of the tragedy.

The Australian migration department, sensitive to the fact that some of the survivors would not want to travel by air again, announced that they would be happy to make alternative arrangements for the families who were going to Australia to live, so that if they preferred they could travel by boat. The Hay family from Warsash near Southampton decided that they would prefer a sea voyage. They were booked on the *Oriana* but before it was ready to leave the vessel suffered a broken propeller which, they were told, would delay their departure for at least another month. Anxious to put their ordeal behind them and get on with their new lives, they decided that they would not wait for the ship to be repaired and instead opted to fly. Trevor Hay recalled the nervousness they all felt about boarding an aircraft again after what had happened but says that the flight they took had its first transit stop in Amsterdam and, having survived this short flight with no mishaps, they were able to continue their journey in a relatively relaxed manner.

Fourteen year old Trevor had lost his prized collection of Southampton footballers' autographs in the fire and, when the club heard about it, manager Ted Bates promised: 'We will see that Trevor gets a new set quickly.' It was planned that he would go to the football club to fetch the autographs himself but, when the *Oriana*'s broken propeller meant that the family would have to go by air after all, there was no time for Trevor to get to the club and so he never got his replacement collection.

Fred and Vera Pragnell took no time at all to decide that if they didn't get on an aircraft very soon they would probably never have the nerve to do so again. They collected their young son Steven, from Ashford hospital where he had spent the night following the accident and, on 9 April boarded another BOAC Boeing 707 flight to Perth with Steven and his sister, Dawn, who was clutching a doll given to her by one of the nursing sisters. With them were several other passengers from Whisky Echo and a reporter, Andrew Fyall, from the *Daily Express*. He flew with the family as far as their first transit stop, Zurich, from where he filed his story, describing how:

> The giant jet, its four Rolls-Royce engines now merely whispering, trundled past the scene of Monday's crash. Only a blackened, twisted skeleton of an engine remained to mark the spot of heroism and death.
>
> I looked the length of the aircraft. Not a single head had turned to look out of the windows. Some people were staring fixedly ahead, others instinctively turned their bodies away from the view of the wreckage.
>
> ...The engines roared into violent life and the plane surged forward. ...Suddenly I was aware that something was different about this flight; something was out of place;

NEARLY EVERYONE WAS TALKING.

...It was 4.25. Foxtrot Golf lifted off halfway along the runway, surged powerfully, almost lazily, into the air.

It banked to port over the gravel pits where the engine of the B.O.A.C. jetliner plummeted to the ground in flames. Only a few passengers looked out.

Eighteen year old student Maryam Entekhavi had also decided to travel as soon as possible. As she said: 'I'm all right and I'm not going to let this interfere with my Easter holiday.'

Another passenger not wanting to delay his departure for a minute longer than he had to was the man who had failed to turn up for his court case the day before. When he had clambered out of the wreckage his details had been taken by the BOAC staff who were trying to build up a list of the survivors. He also telephoned his sister, the only one of his family to have a telephone, and told her that he was all right and that he still intended to go to Australia.[2] Having now become a fugitive the police had been alerted to the fact and, when a policeman at Heathrow spotted his name on the list of survivors and an address in the same northern town from where he had come, he contacted the address and discovered that it was not his home but was that of the travel agent's office from where he had bought his ticket.[3] Becoming very suspicious the police also discovered that he had been booked to take a Qantas flight to Sydney[4] on 9 April and, as a survivor from the previous day, had been invited to wait for his flight in the VIP lounge. Fifteen minutes before the departure of the flight he was arrested there. He was taken back to his home town by police where he appeared in court, pleading guilty to the charge of indecent assault. The prosecuting counsel, Alan Jacks, said:

His whereabouts became known as a result of the Boeing 707 which crashed while taking off for Australia. [He] was given some publicity in the Press.

Detective Constable Frederick Farley told the court:

There was no real intention of emigrating. He only bought the airline tickets as a direct result of these court proceed-

ings. His wife and his family knew nothing about his desire
to go abroad.

The chairwoman of the Bench, Miss E.S. Riley-Lord, told him
that she thought he had been under a great strain and added:

> You have had an experience that has left you in some degree
> of shock.[5]

At Heathrow work had begun to move the wreckage of the
aircraft to a less visible location. The sight of it did not inspire
confidence in any of the airlines using the airport and so the
main part of Whisky Echo was lifted off the runway and taken
back to the BOAC engineering base where it was placed behind
the hangars. Although it could not be seen so easily from the
ground it was still very visible to any passengers who looked
out of the window whenever their flight took-off or landed over
the eastern side of the airport.

Reg Findlay, who worked for BOAC and had witnessed the
stricken jet landing on 8 April, took photos while it remained
behind the hangars, some of which he has kindly allowed the
author to use in this book.

Josephine Pole had just joined BOAC, working in the Number
1 Hangar – Stores Dispatch and had also seen the aircraft land.
She recalled that, even from a distance, it was quite clear that the
inside of the aircraft was a charred mess.

Robin Johnson, another airline employee who had witnessed
the incident, remembered being very concerned about the
length of time that the wreckage was left behind the hangar
while Colin Smith, who had watched the aircraft land from the
roof of BOAC's Technical Block A, went to see the burnt remains
and wished he hadn't:

> After inspecting the wreckage the next day I resolved never
> to visit another accident unless in the line of duty (and I
> haven't).

The morning after the accident, Whisky Echo's No. 2 engine was
found by Royal Navy frogmen, diving in the muddy water of
the gravel pit in Thorpe. It had sunk to the bottom of the pit and

was stuck in the gravel. According to one of the divers it was 'like diving into a bowl of custard'. It took the frogmen until late afternoon to free it and bring it to the bank but the ground was so soft around the edge of the pit that they weren't able to get the engine onto dry land. It was reported in the local newspaper, the *Staines and Egham News*, that Army and Navy personnel planned to:

> ...float the engine on inflatable cushions and tow it across the water to more solid ground from where they would be able to winch it onto a lorry.

It eventually took two days to get the engine out of the water and it was then transferred to a BOAC hangar at Heathrow where the low pressure compressor was removed and sent to Rolls-Royce in Derby. The rest of the engine went to the Royal Aircraft Establishment, in Farnborough, Hampshire, where it was stripped by a team from Rolls-Royce.

As well as the Board of Trade enquiry, BOAC conducted a full investigation itself. The airline's chief engineer, Charles Abell, suggested that perhaps the engine malfunction had been because of a bird strike. He thought it was a possibility if a mechanical breakdown was discounted and said that its recorded 13,000 flying hours meant it was one of the airline's younger engines. Regarding the similarities with the accident to Whisky Echo the previous year in Honolulu he was also quoted as saying:

> All four engines were changed after the previous incident and none of them were the same engines. Since then all the engines in that aircraft and all the other 707s have been modified as a result of that previous incident.
>
> The indications we have got so far are that this is an entirely different type of incident to the one at Honolulu.

The investigations, led by Principal Inspector Norman Head of the Board of Trade and John Boulding, BOAC Inspector of Accidents, would show that, contrary to Charles Abell's assertion, the causes of both incidents were, in fact, quite similar.

Two days after the accident, on Wednesday 10 April, the number 1 shift of BEA engineering staff, amounting to forty-six men, wrote and signed the following letter. They addressed it to Mr Gordon-Burge, Head of the Air Safety Branch, their own manager Mr McLean, the secretary of the British Airline Pilots Association and Mr M. Barnes, the Member of Parliament for Brentford and Chiswick:

B.O.A.C. Boeing 707 Fire: 8th, April 1968.

As eye-witnesses of the B.O.A.C. 707 fire at London Airport, we the undersigned feel morally compelled to register in the strongest of terms the following complaints against the Airport Fire Fighting Service afforded to the above mentioned aircraft.

1). It seems incomprehensible that only <u>two</u> appliances were immediately available when the aircraft came to a halt, in view of the fact that the aircraft was <u>positively</u> <u>on</u> <u>fire</u> before landing.

2). Inadequacy of equipment available: The aforementioned appliances made minimal impression on the fire, the pressure of their hoses being farcical, and under less tragic circumstances would have been comical.

When CO_2 was applied to the fire, results looked encouraging, then the appliance <u>ran</u> <u>out</u> <u>of</u> <u>CO_2.</u> and the blaze took fresh-hold.

Negligible protective clothing. – NO asbestos suits.

3). Doubt as to the disposition and guidance of forces fighting the blaze, e.g. the initial attack was directed at an area near the 'tail-fin'.

4). Why only one CO_2 appliance at the blaze initially?

5). Suspect lack of adequate communication and liaison; the aircraft <u>was</u> on fire, not assumed to be.

If it did land on a different runway to the one initially envisaged, is this adequate reason for it to be attended to, by two appliances only?

We wish to state emphatically that we direct <u>no</u> criticism at the firemen, but consider that in 1968, at the busiest Airport in Europe, the equipment at their disposal is flagrantly inadequate to deal with a conflagration of the size encountered on 8.4.68., especially taking into account the fact that aircraft of the 'Jumbo-Jet' size are a possibility in the very near-future.

The 707 seems beyond the Airport Fire Service's capabilities.

It is ironic that two days after the BEA engineers wrote and signed this damning document, another was being written about the same event but in completely different terms. Raymond M. Hill, Chief Engineer and General Manager, and Ethan N. Carter, Fire Prevention Engineer, both of the City of Los Angeles Department of Fire, sent the following letter to the Ministry of Aviation Chief Fire Service Officer in London:

The air crash and fire involving a BOAC Boeing 707, which occurred in your country last week, has aroused an unusual amount of interest among us in the fire service. The actions taken by the crew and your rescue people are indeed commendable.

May we sir, be furnished with a document or report of your findings which will more clearly tell us just what happened? We would like especially to have particulars as to actions taken after the plane came to rest; those effective actions which may be emulated by our crash-rescue crews if a similar incident should occur here.

When the results of the enquiry into the Whisky Echo tragedy were finally published the following year, the role of the emergency services was one of the areas that was covered extensively. The members of the investigation team were so disturbed by the shortcomings they uncovered, that a large section of the final report was devoted to the facilities provided at Heathrow and focused, primarily, on the airport fire service. There is no record of any further correspondence from the Los Angeles Fire Department.

***

Having left St George's hospital, Mark Wynter spent a very busy few days at the home of his agent, Ian Bevan. Mark had decided that he would fly to Melbourne the following week and, in the meantime, had lots to do. Both his wedding suit and his musical arrangements had been destroyed in the fire and had to be replaced quickly. His tasks were made more difficult by having one of his legs in plaster and needing to use a walking stick to move around. He still intended to fulfil his cabaret engagement in Melbourne and had decided that his wedding would go ahead on 19 April even if he hadn't managed to get rid of the plaster by then. Ian arranged for a tailor to come to his flat and measure Mark for a new suit, and new wedding rings had to be chosen as the box containing those originally picked had also been lost. This flurry of activity helped to take Mark's mind off the horror of the accident and he realized how lucky he had been to get through it all relatively unscathed. He says that Ian Bevan was an absolutely wonderful host and he was very well looked after during the week he stayed with him.

When he eventually arrived at Heathrow, complete with new suit and new wedding rings, he was surprised and pleased to find that BOAC had upgraded his ticket to first class. The flight was uneventful and Mark was reunited with his fiancée in Melbourne. His photo appeared on the front page of Melbourne newspaper, *The Herald* on 17 April showing him having his 'London made wedding suit fitted by Melbourne tailor, Eugenio Nicolini'. The article continued:

> He has been fighting against odds to get to the church on time for his marriage to Melbourne dancer, Janeece Corlass, 24, on Friday.
>
> But now he says he'll be standing at the altar when his fiancée walks down the aisle at 5 p.m.
>
> 'Few people will know what I've been through to get to this wedding' he said at his hotel today.
>
> Mark, 25, still has a foot in plaster from injuries in the Boeing 707 airliner crash at London Airport 10 days ago.

That same day Mark was astonished to receive a phone call from London. It was from *Daily Mirror* journalist, Donald Zec, informing him that when the items salvaged from the wreckage of Whisky Echo had been examined and catalogued, it was discovered that two boxes belonging to Mark had been found. One contained his fountain pen, the birthday present from his fan club, while the other had the two wedding rings he had lost. Not only had all three items been found, they were all still intact. Although Mark no longer uses the pen now, he still has it and, when Ian Bevan flew out to Australia the day before Mark and Janeece's wedding, to be Mark's best man, he brought with him the two wedding rings which the couple used in their marriage ceremony.

For the Cooper family the nightmare was still not over. At a time when they should have been well on their way to Perth, Brian Cooper was given the task that every father prays he will never have to face; he had to formally identify the body of his little girl.

When Shirley was released from hospital the family went, not to Perth, but back to their family in Southampton to arrange Jacky's funeral. She was buried in Millbrook cemetery next to her paternal grandmother, Eva, who had died the year before.

Brian and Shirley didn't know what they should do about going to Australia. They had been looking forward to their new life for such a long time but couldn't decide if it would be better to remain in England, now that Jacky was no longer with them, or if they should go ahead with the original plan. Eventually they turned to Brian's father, Thomas, for his advice. He told them that they should stick to their original plan and emigrate, reasoning that they would not feel any better, and life would not be any easier, if they remained in England. They decided that he was right and, two weeks after their ordeal on Whisky Echo, boarded another flight bound for Australia. They managed to get as far as Zurich but had been so traumatized by the accident that they found they could not go any further by air and so left the flight in Switzerland and made their way back to Southampton by train and boat. A sea passage was then arranged for them and they sailed for the port of Fremantle via Las Palmas and Cape Town.

In York during the week following the tragedy, Jane Harrison's funeral was arranged by her father and sister. It was held in St George's Catholic Church close to Sue's home and was attended, not only by Jane's family and friends, but by representatives of BOAC as well, including the airline's chairman, Sir Giles Guthrie, Flight Operations Director, Captain Frank Walton, Cabin Crew Manager, Stan Bruce and Jane's Flight Stewardess, Penny Casson. Sir Giles spoke to Sue after the church service and she remembers that he was extremely upset and close to tears.

Margaret Jessop was still in Rome and was not aware that Jane had died until later so was not at her funeral but her other school friends, Kay Golightly and Sheila Walkington, met up at a nearby public house, along with one of Jane's former boyfriends, Ian Cartlidge,[6] and the three went to the church together but did not attend the burial in nearby Fulford cemetery. Kay recalled that, as it was the final week of Lent, according to Roman Catholic tradition, there were no flowers at the funeral. She was upset at not being able to take flowers for Jane and so returned to the cemetery after Easter to put some on her friend's grave; something she still does to this day.

Chapter 8

Replacements, Investigations and Reports

While the official investigations into the cause of the accident to Whisky Echo were set in motion, BOAC began to consider how it was going to replace its wrecked aircraft.

On 10 April William Davis, financial editor of *The Guardian* reported:

> I gather that the hull of Whisky Echo, the jet which crashed at London Airport on Monday, was insured for £2.2 millions. It means a hefty bill for City underwriters, but the chairman of Lloyds yesterday sent a telegram to Sir Giles Guthrie, chairman of BOAC, asking him to convey his appreciation of 'the crew's magnificent airmanship' to Captain Taylor. It was a genuine tribute, but, of course, underwriters were also lucky to avoid still heavier liability.

The airline had set to work immediately after the accident to find a replacement and, on 19 April, the staff magazine, *BOAC News*, reported that:

> Negotiations have been concluded to replace Whiskey Echo with a new 707. This is one of three ordered a year ago by Saturn Airways, an American non-scheduled carrier.
>
> The agreement with Saturn enables BOAC to receive the new 707 jet in June, four months before a standard 707 would be available from Boeing, and more than a year before it could provide one to BOAC's special requirements.
>
> The aircraft is expected to be in service by late July after it

has been adapted to BOAC passenger and flight deck requirements.

As with the last three 707 cargo jets from Boeing, it will be powered by Pratt and Whitney engines. Government approval has been granted.

***

Despite the severity of the fire, the Epsilon Flight Data Acquisition system – the black box flight recorder – on board Whisky Echo had been located in the wreckage of the tail and was found to be intact. Its only damage seemed to be a degree of blackening from the smoke and the cassette containing all the data was able to be played without any problems. From the black box it was possible to establish the exact duration of the flight, which was three minutes and thirty-two seconds, the fact that the 707 reached an altitude of slightly less than 3,000 feet above the level of Heathrow, and that its maximum speed during the flight was 225 knots. It also disclosed that when it landed it was on a heading of 050°M and continued on this heading for approximately twenty-five seconds before turning to heading 035°M where it remained for the rest of the recording, less than half a minute later. The change in heading meant that the aircraft had veered slightly left of the centre of runway 05R but its position had no bearing on the subsequent events. Although cockpit voice recorders were in operation in 1968, their use was not mandatory. Whisky Echo did not have one fitted and so that evidence, now regarded as vital in aircraft accidents, was not available to the investigators, although all the crew members made very full statements after their escape from the wreckage.

The investigation took almost a year to complete and the report into the enquiry was published in August 1969. It was very detailed and was divided into three sections:

(A) The engine failure and resulting fire.

(B) Matters relating to fire drills in the air.

(C) Evacuation and survival aspects, including the part played by the airport fire and rescue services.

The engine in the No. 2 position, a Rolls-Royce Conway 508 – engine number 5097 – had run for a total of 14,917 hours from new. Constructed in 1961, it was older than the aircraft itself. It had had a complete overhaul in the spring of 1965 but two months later was taken out of service because of a vibration which, on investigation, was found to have been caused by metal fatigue leading to the failure of a stage 8 high pressure compressor blade. Having been repaired and returned to service it performed well for the next two years but was then removed again because of flame tube deterioration and was sent back to the BOAC Engine Overhaul facility in Treforest, south Wales where, as part of the repairs, the low pressure compressor was stripped and overhauled. The No. 5 wheel which failed on 8 April was an original component of this low pressure compressor but, according to the standard procedures for this work, the engineers were not required to check for cracks which would indicate the onset of metal fatigue.

The engine was bench tested on 22 November 1967 but was initially rejected after several runs because of excessive vibration close to the high pressure compressor. Although the level of vibration fell within the acceptable limits of the engine manufacturer, BOAC had amended the limits for engines fitted to its aircraft and these were more stringent than those of Rolls-Royce. However, after more analysis the engine was finally released and declared serviceable.

During the enquiry into the causes of the accident on 8 April, an error in the way the results of the vibration test figures had been calculated, came to light. The Chief Inspector of Accidents at the Board of Trade, Captain V.A.M. Hunt was concerned enough about this error to contact Walter Tye at the Air Registration Board to tell him what he had found. He stressed that this was, in no way, directly connected with the accident but he wanted to point out that the way in which the figures had been calculated suggested that the vibration was of a low pressure order rather than high pressure and that, if this had been known, it was probable that the engine wouldn't have been

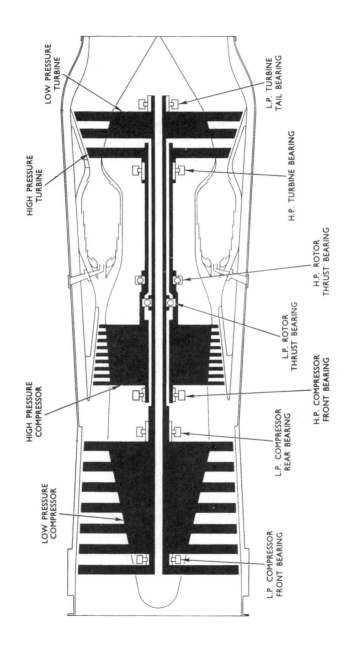

ROLLS-ROYCE CONWAY ENGINE – MAIN ROTATING ASSEMBLY. THE PART THAT FAILED IN WHISKY ECHO'S NUMBER 2 ENGINE WAS THE 5TH STAGE LOW PRESSURE COMPRESSOR WHEEL.

Diagram courtesy of Captain E.D. 'Wyn' Fieldson

released but would have been stripped down for investigation, as there had been concerns about the high pressure compressors at that time.

Since Captain Hunt did not believe that this had anything to do with the accident on 8 April, he did not make note of it in the official report. It would, however, seem logical to assume, since this had no effect on the accident, that regardless of whether or not these additional investigations had been made, the No. 5 low pressure compressor wheel would have failed anyway at some point and potentially caused an accident to whichever aircraft the engine had been fitted.

Having been released as serviceable, however, it was fitted to another 707 where it remained for a further 1,415 hours before being removed again for a modification to the turbine seals. Following this modification, on 5 April 1968, it became No. 2 engine on the port wing of Whisky Echo.

When it was recovered from the gravel pit in Thorpe, after the accident, and examined by the working party from Rolls-Royce, their report was summarized in six points:

1. The primary failure within engine No. 5097 was of the 5th stage low pressure compressor wheel.

2. This wheel had failed in fatigue at the run out radius of the wheel web with the rim.

3. The failures of the 4-5 and 5-6 low pressure compressor spacers were secondary to the 5th stage wheel failure.

4. The failure of the low pressure compressor casing, the engine cowlings, low pressure compressor blades and stators, and the low pressure fuel pipe retaining sleeve were all secondary to the 5th stage wheel failure.

5. All other damage was considered to be due to impact with the water, or associated with recovery of the pod and pylon from the gravel pit.

6. Fire damage to the engine was confined to minor sooting and slight paint blistering in random areas. The fire was

secondary to the wheel failure and loss of the low pressure fuel feed pipe from the disconnect platform to the Nash backing pump.

Although the fire on the aircraft was the main cause of its destruction, it was the failure of the No. 5 low pressure compressor wheel, that was held to blame for the fire. The enquiry report divided the account of the fire into two stages. The first dealt with the position immediately after the compressor failure and the second following the engine falling from the wing.

It was found that when the compressor wheel broke up it burst through its casing. This pushed the main fuel feed pipe out of alignment and disconnected it. Fuel was then being pumped at a rate of 50 gallons per minute (approximately 150 kilos per minute) through the broken pipe into the damaged compressor and onwards to the combustion area where it ignited immediately. Because such a lot of the engine cowling had been destroyed by the broken compressor casing, and had fallen off, the fire extinguishers located within the engine were ineffectual and the fire continued to burn at a fierce rate. Had the fuel shut-off valve been closed it should have been possible to extinguish the fire but this was not done. Because the fire had continued to burn in such a ferocious manner the engine pylon was severely weakened and, when it gave way completely, the engine fell off the wing. Following the loss of the engine and, with the fuel booster pump continuing to supply the fire with fuel through the broken pipe, the fire intensified. It was burning from forward of the wing's leading edge and the flames were sweeping back over the wing towards the tail. When the aircraft landed, the direction of the fire changed, following the use of the reverse thrust, and flames began licking underneath the wing and in towards the fuselage. The fire got worse after the aircraft stopped as the fuel booster pumps were still operating for about twenty seconds longer. Then the electrical circuits were destroyed by the fire which cut off the power to the pumps and stopped them from delivering any more fuel. By this stage the flames and smoke were so bad that it became clear that what had been an emergency landing was now a major incident. With the fire burning so fiercely a series of explosions occurred, releasing fuel from the tanks in the port wing. The main focus at that point had to be the prevention of the fire reaching the fuel tanks in the starboard wing which were still intact and contained enough kerosene to cause a disastrous explosion if the fire was not contained.

Although the investigators were of the opinion that, had the fuel shut-off valve been closed, it should have been possible to extinguish the fire, there were others who disagreed. It was only seconds into the flight when the cockpit crew heard the bang and felt the aircraft lurch and they had no idea at that time that there was a fire taking hold. They had commenced their Engine Failure drill which, at that time, did not include pulling the fire shut-off handle, and it was only when Geoff Moss discovered that the wing was on fire that the Engine Fire drill was started, by which time the fire was so well established that it was not just burning because it had a supply of fuel from the booster pump. The severing of the main fuel feed pipe had already allowed an enormous amount of fuel to escape which, many believe, was enough to keep the fire burning anyway, even if the pump had been switched off.

As we have already seen in Chapter 4, the cockpit drills that were in force at the time of the accident added to the confusion in the cockpit during the short time that Whisky Echo was in the air. The report made reference to this and quoted parts of each of the drills – Engine Failure and Engine Fire – in a horizontal layout that compared some of the steps that had to be taken in each situation. It emphasized the point that the first phase of each of the drills had to be done from memory without any repetition against a checklist whilst the second phase was done with the aid of a checklist. It is hard to see why this method was used but the report stated that BOAC had compiled these drills using those of the aircraft manufacturer and other airlines operating the same aircraft type. Where BOAC differed was in allocating a task to a specific crew member by the use of a single letter to signify whose task it was, e.g. E – engineer etc. It was the airline's policy not to change any procedures such as these drills in case the changes confused staff already used to them. They would only do so if they found that their existing procedures were seriously flawed and the investigation into this accident led BOAC to make significant changes, the main one being that the two drills were combined, forming a new one which was called the 'Engine Fire or Severe Failure Drill'. It was also felt that the operation of the fire shut-off handle should be confirmed by the pilot. It was the responsibility of the engineer but, the report stated, it could only be done if his seat belt was very loose. It was also reported that:

> Since the accident the operations flying manual has been revised to state more specifically the procedure to be followed. It now requires that after completion of the drill the check list shall be read from the beginning and that if the nature of the emergency prevents the list being read in the normal manner,[1] the Flight Engineer, once the drill has been called for, will perform and check the items himself by reference to the check list and that whenever a drill has been performed in this way it shall be checked by a normal reading of the check list from the beginning as soon as possible.

Perhaps significantly, in view of the fact that Captain Geoff Moss had reached over to operate a switch and had ordered Cliff Taylor to use runway 05R when it was offered, the report also stated:

> The Route Check Captain's duties are designed to ensure that agreed standards of operation are maintained. The Captain under check operates the section concerned exactly in accordance with his normal operating procedures. The Check Captain may not request a particular procedure and in general is expected to be as unobtrusive as possible.

It did also say, however, that Cliff Taylor had given Geoff Moss the briefing he would normally have given to the third pilot[2] which was to 'act as an extra pair of eyes, both inside and outside the cockpit, to advise the operating crew of any unusual circumstances'. Apart from reaching for the switch to turn off the warning horn at the same time as engineer Thomas Hicks, it would seem that this is exactly what Geoff Moss did.

During the early part of the investigation a letter was sent to Jim Templeton at the Air Registration Board from the Chief Investigating Officer, E. Newton, on behalf of the Chief Inspector of Accidents, Captain V.A.M. Hunt, calling into question the suitability of the engine fire control switches in the 707 cockpit. He was concerned that the pull out switch which armed the fire bottle circuit and also closed the emergency fuel and hydraulic oil shut off valves was very light in use and could easily be pushed in accidentally when reaching for other switches. The report did not highlight this apparent flaw but, in view of the fact that the switch moved only about half an inch when pulled out, did say that from the flight engineer's position, it was not easy to see whether or not the switch had been operated and that the captain and first officer had a better view of it. The investigators seemed to think that the switch itself was not conspicuous enough to be immediately noticed by any of the crew in the middle of a tense emergency situation and that this was a problem.

The evidence about the ease with which the switch could be inadvertently pushed back in, must lead one to speculate that perhaps this is what happened in Whisky Echo. The flight engineer had the impression that he had pulled the shut-off switch as part of the fire drill, an impression which was shared by the first officer. Perhaps he had done so but it had then been knocked back in again while the crew were struggling to keep the aircraft in the air. There is divided opinion about whether or not the switch might have been kicked by one of the three members of the crew who left via the cockpit window and used the escape rope to reach the ground. Reaching the window involved a certain amount of climbing over seats and instruments and it is possible, some say, that, in their haste, a leg or a foot may have knocked against the switch. Others think it unlikely to have been a possible cause for the switch to have been pushed back in. It clearly was in the 'IN' position when recovered from the wreckage and the emergency fuel and hydraulic oil shut-off valves were open. The enquiry found that although Geoff Moss had been briefed by Cliff Taylor to keep a watch out for anything unusual he had not paid particular attention to the fire drill as he thought it more important to keep Captain Taylor informed about the progress of the fire itself and was looking out of the window towards the blazing wing. The report stated that he had not noticed that the fire shut-off handle had not been pulled and, when he looked back into the cockpit:

> ...the engine had fallen away and consequently the warning light in the fire handle had gone out – so that his attention was not drawn in that direction.

Since none of the cockpit crew was aware that the engine had fallen off until they were on the ground, Geoff Moss could not have known that the light had gone out because the engine was no longer there and would have assumed it was out because the fire switch had been pulled, as did the other members of the crew.

The accident report also said that:

> From the weight of evidence it seems that the fire bell did not ring because the First Officer, after hearing the under-carriage horn start to sound, misidentified the action required and was pressing the fire bell cancel button at the instant when the bell would have started to ring. Therefore consideration has been given to the possible effect this may have had on the performance of the drills. No definite con-clusion can be reached but there is a possibility that the Flight Engineer would have been alerted to a greater extent to the need to start with the memory items of the fire drill if the first action he was required to perform had been the can-cellation of the warning bell.

Regarding the actions of the First Officer, the report called attention to the fact that although the Flight Engineer had told him that the first part of the fire drill had been completed, if the First Officer had read the check items back himself, it would have made no difference to what happened as: 'a check of the fire shut-off handle would not have been included'.

In relation to the actions of the cockpit crew the report concluded:

The First Officer's cancellation of the fire bell instead of the undercarriage warning horn prevented the fire bell from ringing.

The closure of the fuel shut-off valve by pulling the fire handle was inadvertently omitted by the Flight Engineer when he carried out the fire drill. The omission was not noticed by the Captain, the First Officer or the Check Captain. The Second Officer[3] was in no position to observe the situation.

The failure to close the fuel shut-off valve permitted the fire to continue.

The BOAC Fire and Engine Overheat or Failure Drills in force at the time were capable of misapplication under stress.

When it came to the events in the cabin, the report criticized the aircraft's escape chute fittings saying that, although BOAC had introduced modifications which would make the operation of the chutes easier, it would be better if they required no special fittings at all and were, therefore, ready for use whenever they might be needed. Of the cabin crew, the investigators had very little to say, except to pay tribute to them. It had been a textbook evacuation and the report praised the cabin staff for the way they prepared the passengers for the emergency landing and evacuation, and for their 'commendable coolness and efficiency throughout'. It was the opinion of the accident investigators that:

It is undoubtedly due to the efforts of the cabin staff that the loss of life was not greater.

Helen Muir, OBE, Professor of Aerospace Psychology at Cranfield University, has made a study of passenger safety in transport aircraft. She says that research shows that one assertive cabin attendant can evacuate passengers quicker than two who are not assertive:

In the accidents where a successful rapid evacuation of all the passengers is achieved, the cabin crew will have managed to control the passengers (despite a fire and the presence of smoke in the cabin) and prevented disorderly behaviour from occurring.

Today the usual ratio of passengers to cabin crew is 50:1. On Whisky Echo the figure was nearly 26:1, and this was supplemented by members of the cockpit crew helping once the aircraft had come to a standstill. What was probably most important was that the crew seems to have had a very positive attitude to getting everyone off as soon as they possibly could. Under the leadership of Neville Davis-Gordon each performed his or her duties in a very professional manner, instructing, informing, assisting and, ultimately, pushing and sometimes physically throwing passengers down the chutes and out of open doorways in their attempts to save them.

It is interesting to note that the report into the enquiry stated that:

> The evidence has shown that the great concern of the passengers to take their small belongings with them tends to block up the gangways.

Professor Muir says of this behaviour:

> Passengers' attachment to their hand luggage has often been observed, with many passengers insisting on taking their personal belongings with them when undertaking an emergency evacuation. It seems the perceived value of the contents obviously outweighs the increased risk they believe they will encounter, by taking it with them.

According to Professor Muir's research, passengers' own motivation can lead either to an orderly evacuation or to a total shambles. In the case of the former, they know that they all have to get off and so behave in a way that allows each person to move as quickly as possible to an escape route to achieve this. Where a disaster in the evacuation occurs it is because the passengers are not thinking of themselves as part of a group, with a common problem, but are regarding the objective of leaving the aircraft as their own individual problem and will often fight other passengers, trample them or break seats to ensure that they can get out, not caring what happens to anyone else.

In any emergency situation aboard an aircraft the mix of passengers must, therefore, have a great influence on whether or not escape is possible. In the case of Whisky Echo it was fortunate that both crew and passengers seem to have been team players; the crew were assertive and quick thinking and the passengers, for the most part, showed very little panic, obeying instructions as quickly as they could and working together to get out as swiftly as possible. In ninety seconds 111 passengers had left the aircraft using two exits over the starboard wing and two of the aircraft's four escape chutes, with only one in use for most of the time. Eight of the ten surviving crew members had escaped using the forward chute and the rope from the cockpit window while the remaining two had climbed down twisted chutes to straighten them; the Flight Engineer at the front and the Steward at the back.

In direct contrast to this accident, was the one which occurred at Manchester airport in 1985 to a British Airtours Boeing 737 bound for Corfu with 131 passengers and six crew on board. The 737 also caught fire when an engine failed on take-off but there the similarity with the Whisky Echo accident ended. Although the passengers on the 737 had over two minutes to leave the aircraft, compared with the ninety seconds for Whisky Echo, and had half of the emergency exits fully functioning, fifty-five passengers died, including two stewardesses, four children and a baby.

Despite most people wanting to escape from a burning aircraft as soon as they possibly can, there are instances where they seem physically unable to do so although they may be perfectly able bodied in normal life. This state, where the person seems to freeze, as in the case of the two women onboard Whisky Echo, is more common than one would suppose and is known as behavioural inaction. Incredibly it is believed that there are more cases of behavioural inaction than of panic. In some cases up to 25 per cent of passengers have been observed doing nothing to save themselves. In contrast others manage to achieve what would, under normal circumstances, be unachievable.

Although simulated emergency situations can include incentives to encourage the participants to behave as if they really were in danger, it would be difficult to actually induce behavioural inaction during an exercise and so the methods for counteracting this phenomenon cannot be fully explored.

When asked what it was that had driven Jane Harrison to go back into the cabin in search of the last passengers still on board, Professor Muir said simply: 'Sheer bravery'.

***

When addressing the problems encountered with the fighting of the fire, the accident investigators made a separate report, attached to the main report as an annex, and based on the results of the Fire and Rescue Service Working Group. This small group was set up under the chairmanship of Mr G. Wilkinson, an inspector of accidents at the AIB and comprised the Chief Officer at Liverpool Fire Brigade, Mr F. Taylor, the Deputy Chief Fire Service Officer at the Board of Trade, Mr J. MacDonald, and associate member of the group, Mr E. Williams, who was Chief Fire Officer for the British Airports Authority. Their conclusions make dismal reading as they catalogue a series of disasters which included delays in being able to give clearance to the fire vehicles to cross live runways due to existing aircraft movements, errors in positioning vehicles, breakdowns in the equipment, and explosions from the aircraft limiting the area in which the vehicles could operate.

As anyone who has ever tried to get a garden bonfire started with a splash of fuel will know, even a very small amount of volatile liquid will instantly produce a relatively large fire. Three and a half minutes after take-off, Whisky Echo had returned to Heathrow with a large amount of the 22,000 kilos of fuel that had been pumped into it before departure, still onboard. Speed was of the essence in bringing the fire under control.

When John Davis in the control tower first operated the crash line it was assumed that Whisky Echo would return to the airport via the same runway it had used when it took off. At that time the rendezvous point for the outside emergency services was on the south-east side of the airport, close to runway 28L. When it became clear that there would be no time to reach 28L and clearance was given for an approach to 05R the ATCO again hit the crash line and changed the rendezvous point to 'North' outside of the main fire station. The change was necessary as the aircraft landed on a runway which ran from the south-west to the north-east. Because of the way in which the airport had been designed it was not ideal as 05R ran across the middle of the airfield and was, for the most part, framed by parallel runways, 28R and 28L to the north and south, which meant that wherever the rendezvous point was, the emergency services would have to cross live runways to reach the scene of the fire.

The two fire appliances that followed the aircraft down the runway were a foam/CO_2 tender and a water tender. The former stopped about seventy feet to the left of, and behind, the port tailplane. The latter parked close by and started to transfer water to the foam tender. Two hand lines were used by firemen to direct the foam towards the fire near to the port rear door. On top of the foam tender was a monitor; a metal tube which looked rather like the barrel of a large gun and could be moved to give the best direction for the foam to be delivered into the fire. The monitor also directed foam towards the rear door. These were the vehicles that had been seen by the BEA engineers and about which they had been so critical.

Not long after it went into operation the monitor was shut down; it was thought to be because of a possible fault in the foam proportioning equipment, the Vactrol unit, which was a cylinder and piston assembly and worked in much the same way as a vacuum-servo braking system. At the same time the offside hand held hose burst and a short delay ensued while it was being replaced. It was noted in the report that these initial attempts to douse the flames were largely inadequate anyway as the foam tender was parked too far away from the fire and the hand held lines were also too far away to make a difference.

It should have been possible to move the foam tender closer to the aircraft but it was revealed that the type of tenders used by the BAA fire service, Nubian TFA 6x6s, could not make foam when underway and, having stopped for foam production, could then not be repositioned.

At about this time further explosions occurred on the aircraft setting fire to the starboard rear chute down which passengers had been escaping. The two hand held lines were used to fight the fire for about four minutes before both tenders ran out of water. The firemen then tried to use the CO_2 supply which amounted to 400 lb but the hose reel became disconnected and the CO_2 escaped into the air without making any useful contribution to putting out the blaze.

After a large explosion caused the aircraft's back to be broken the main part of the fire fighting force arrived, having been delayed for approximately thirty to forty-five seconds while waiting for clearance to cross 28R as one inbound aircraft landed and two more were instructed to overshoot. When the other vehicles did arrive a foam tender was positioned on the grass, level with the nose of the aircraft, and about sixty-five feet from the runway's edge. The water tender pulled alongside and began transferring water but as soon as the hand held lines were deployed, in a repeat of what had happened at the rear of the aircraft, one of them also burst and had to be replaced, incurring yet another delay of about a minute. As the tender was so far from the aircraft anyway it was not possible to use the monitor which was out of range. Ten minutes after Whisky Echo had come to a standstill on the runway these two tenders had used up their supplies of foam and water.

There were, of course, hydrants to connect the vehicles to a mains water supply but to do this a hose-laying vehicle had to be there. At the time of the landing this vehicle was on a familiarization exercise in the central area and its occupants did not hear any radio messages about attending the fire. They did, however, see the thick pall of smoke and went to its source as soon as they could, arriving about three minutes after Whisky Echo. They connected two hoses to the nearest hydrant and laid them as far as the foam tender on the grass but as the water began to flow through the hoses the pressure blew the coupling joint on one of them and the water had to be switched off. The other hose coupling held but, as the firemen were working on the broken coupling, this hose was not connected to an appliance and was only of use when one of the crew attached it to the foam tender near to the tailplane which had used up its onboard supply of water. The rogue coupling was finally attached to another hydrant but only after the hose was man-handled by the crew over a distance of about 300 feet which took them about eight minutes to do. By then another four tenders had used up all their onboard water and for approximately one minute no foam or water was being directed onto the fire at all.

A Cardox CO_2 truck arrived at the nose of the aircraft a little after the other vehicles and discharged gas into the fire on what remained of the port wing. Just as it appeared that it was under control the supply of CO_2 was exhausted and with no functioning foam tender available to take over, the fire once more sprang into life and spread rapidly.

One foam tender at the front of the aircraft did manage to prevent the fire spreading to the starboard wing where the fuel tanks were still intact and thereby prevented another huge explosion.

Although two firemen wearing breathing apparatus attended the fire and made repeated attempts to get on board, they were driven back by the heat and only later managed to enter through the starboard rear door.

The London Fire Brigade and the London Ambulance Service from the surrounding areas also attended the fire. Both services arrived at the rendezvous point 'North' about seven minutes after the aircraft landed and five minutes after they had been called to attend. Despite their timely response to the call there was a delay before they left the rendezvous point to go to 05R, accompanied by BAA police. It emerged in the accident report that there was a disagreement between the BAA and the LFB:

> The LFB and BAA do not agree as to the reasons for this delay. The senior LFB officer with the first attendance of the

LFB left his appliance and entered the BAA watchroom. He maintains that he was informed that a Boeing 707 aircraft with 131 persons[4] on board had caught fire on emergency landing and its port wing was alight; the fire was under control and his appliances were to remain at the rendezvous point. In view of the apparent size of the fire, however, he decided to go forward with his appliances. The BAA watchroom attendant recorded in the log that the LFB were 'on station' at 1537 hrs.[5] and given all information regarding the accident. At 1538 hrs. a signal was received from the senior BAA officer at the scene of the accident requesting that the LFB should be sent forward. The LFB were informed and left under BAA police escort. When further LFB appliances arrived at the rendezvous point, they were held up awaiting escort vehicles to take them to the accident, as all the available BAA police vehicles had departed with the first LFB contingent. In the event, off duty BAA firemen acted as guides and directed the appliances to the scene of the accident. The LFB attendance comprised 22 vehicles and provided water, manpower and equipment in support of the BAA fire service.

In its findings the working group examined many other things including the number of fire fighting personnel available on 8 April and the means by which they were made aware that a major incident was in progress.

Their report revealed that there were a total of twenty-six fire fighters on duty at the time of the accident. Of these only twenty-one responded to the first emergency call. One was in the stores at the time they were initially alerted and was late in arriving, one had been allocated the duty of watchroom attendant, yet another – a crew member from one of the foam tenders – was not available due to having been rostered as the acting duty driver, while the other two were on the hose-layer in the centre of the airport making a familiarization trip.

Although John Davis had correctly hit the crash line as soon as he could, this did not immediately inform everyone of what was happening. The crash line was a unidirectional line from the control tower to the fire service watchroom. When the button was hit it turned on a light in the watchroom and switched on alarm bells. The information given by ATC on the crash line was monitored by the airport switchboard, the fire service sub station watchroom, in the centre of the airport, and the BAA police but the way in which the information was relayed to all concerned was by attendants in the watchrooms being first alerted by the bells and then announcing the emergency over loudspeakers. The main station attendant then had to contact the LFB and LAS by telephone. It was not the most efficient of systems and was regarded by the working group as being:

...time-consuming and ponderous. Thought should be given to alerting the LFB at the same time as the BAA fire service. The use of the crash bells to alert personnel for all callouts is highly undesirable. The crash alarm signal should be quite distinctive and different to that used to signify routine and domestic turnouts. Ideally, it should only be heard in connection with aircraft accidents and ground incidents.

The communications problems did not end here. In addition to the rather slow method of informing all concerned about an accident or an impending incident, some of the emergency services also had their own radio systems which allowed them to communicate within their own sections but not with each other. The BAA sections using radio communications were the fire service, the police and the MT and marshalling section with their own VHF frequency. The Metropolitan Police, the LFB and the LAS had another VHF frequency while the ATC Ground Movement Controller had yet another. The working group found that:

At the time of the accident there were twenty-one different VHF frequencies operated by seven separate agencies concerned with fire fighting and rescue operations at Heathrow, but no provision has been made for direct communications between the various authorities or for monitoring other services' frequencies, apart from a selective calling (SELCAL) facility provided between some of the

BAA fire service vehicles and the GMC position in ATC, whereby actuation of a switch by the fire officer illuminates a light and sounds a buzzer in ATC. A switch is then made in ATC which allows direct R/T contact between the GMC and the fire vehicle. When the fire officer wishes to sever contact the Selcal switch has to be reset by ATC. If this is not done, GMC signals can saturate the fire service frequency.

It would be hard to imagine a more complicated and potentially confusing system.

When the Fire and Rescue Service Working Group completed its study in March 1969 it made eleven points in its conclusion. These included the fact that the number of vehicles, supplies and personnel was in excess of those required by the airport licence; the fire service prevented the starboard wing fuel tank from exploding; and the fire service personnel were given more training than that which was recommended. It did, however, point out that the deployment of the fire appliances, 'with the exception of the Cardox unit, was poor'; the attendance of the LFB was delayed due to 'poor communications and inadequate liaison'; the communications networks of the various agencies 'require integrating and rationalising'; the airport fire service required more 'frequent and realistic "hot" fire practices'; the faults to the hydrants at Heathrow needed to be 'rectified without delay' and that more foam liquid should be taken to the scenes of fires to 'allow the sustained production of foam'. Worryingly it also stated that:

The level of manning of the BAA fire service, although well in excess of the licensing requirements, was below that necessary to carry out fire fighting and rescue duties efficiently and simultaneously at a major conflagration.

The report concluded with the recommendation that:

A broadly based working party, including members from Home Office Fire Service Department, local authorities, BOT and BAA, should be formed to study and report on the problems of aircraft fire and rescue operations. Their terms of reference should include liaison between airport and local authorities, the siting of fire stations, manning (including command structure), fire and rescue equipment, media scales, the training of firemen and the scale of ambulance cover.

Just one week after the accident report was published in August 1969, a memo, written by D.F. Peel, Director, Aerodromes Technical Directorate, noted that:

Improvements have been made to the Crash Telephone Emergency System.

Action is in hand by B.A.A. to provide a new Console desk at Heathrow Headquarters Fire Station; recording equipment will be included.

Action is in progress with the London Fire Brigade to give them early warning of any potential accident. Their Control System at Wembley will be alerted from Heathrow by the emergency button. Appliances will be turned out and the relevant details passed to them as soon as possible.

The internal Fire Station alarm has been modified and the alarm bells have been replaced by a siren for use only in an aircraft accident of 'full emergency'.

The vehicles equipment and quantities of extinguishing agents provided at Heathrow are in excess of those required by our licensing standards and of those recommended by BOAC. B.A.A. have on order new and larger vehicles with more up to date equipment.

As a result of the failure of the hydrant couplings, B.A.A. have made arrangements with their Airport Works Department for improvements in the maintenance and better inspection of the hydrants.

The cause of the hose failures is not certain but improved equipment is being provided which should reduce the risk of future failure.

...Additional 'hot fire' training is now carried out on a regular basis by retaining crews on duty over-time to avoid depletion of the normal fire cover. Better fire ground facilities have been provided. Discussions are proceeding with the Board of Trade Chief Fire Service Officer on the possibility of making special arrangements to attend the Board's School for intensive training.

Pending an increase in the B.A.A. Police complement, the emergency arrangements will now provide for a marshaller's radio van to report to the rendezvous point to assist the police in guiding vehicles to an accident.

The memo also announced the setting up of the 'broadly based working party' recommended in the report of the Fire and Rescue Service Working Group. In addition it stated:

There is no doubt that the tactics employed on this occasion were poor. However, past and subsequent performances of the Heathrow Fire Service suggest that this was an isolated case.

If this was to be believed, it would suggest that either everyone involved in the previous incidents had been extremely lucky or the airport authorities, in reviewing and upgrading their systems as described, were overreacting. It was obvious that the systems and equipment did need to be replaced and so it was unlikely to have been a case of overreacting but it had taken the Whisky Echo tragedy to alert the authorities to this fact. Had the aircraft not caught fire that April afternoon and the improvements not been made so quickly after the accident there may have been an even bigger catastrophe when the first Boeing 747s and their vastly increased payloads began arriving at Heathrow airport in January 1970.

***

The purpose of an air accident investigation is to discover what went wrong so that improvements can be made to ensure that such accidents do not happen again. It is not concerned with looking into the hearts and minds of the people who fly the aircraft, care for the passengers or man the emergency services and there may have been many explanations for what happened to Whisky Echo.

Although there were clearly a number of serious problems with the emergency services' equipment and a lot of it, and their associated procedures, needed to be updated, it was not thought that these shortcomings would have made any difference to the ultimate outcome. The report of the working group considered it 'doubtful' that, even if the fire fighting vehicles had been better positioned at the accident site, more lives would have been saved. At the time of the accident a fire resistant overall was being developed which could be worn over a fireman's normal clothing but even if it had been available then, the ferocious heat from the fire and the series of explosions on the aircraft would have prevented anyone getting on board until it was too late to save the four women and the little girl.

The pilots and engineer who were rostered to operate the flight to Zurich on 8 April were very different in character but all of them were highly experienced aircrew. The eldest, Check Captain Moss, was fifty years old and had a very forceful personality; the youngest was thirty year old Acting First Officer John Hutchinson who, despite his youth, had 4,120 flying hours to his credit, 680 having been flown on Boeing 707s. In between were the other three men; Francis Kirkland with 5,496 hours, 2,829 of which were on 707 aircraft, Cliff Taylor, a quiet, private man but with more flying hours than anyone else on the crew and Thomas Hicks, the Flight Engineer. It is interesting to note that he had a total of 6,436 flying hours but only 191 of them were on Boeing 707 aircraft. In fact, although he had been free from duty for the previous twenty-two days, 52 of those hours were shown as having been flown during the thirty days before the accident. He was, therefore, less used to the aircraft type than the others but was, nonetheless, not a novice when it came to flying.

With a five-man crew, the cockpit was full that day and, although it is possible that some of them may have flown together before, it was unlikely that they knew each other very well, as crew rostering did not allow for crews that always flew together, unlike RAF crews during the war.

The flight was planned to be a short one; it took approximately an hour and a half to reach Zurich, and, although it wasn't completely full, the aircraft was carrying 115 passengers and eleven crew.

Because Geoff Moss was on board to check Cliff Taylor, there may have been a feeling amongst the rest of the crew that they also were being watched. It was not Captain Moss's function to do so, and there is absolutely no suggestion that he behaved in anything other than a proper manner, but he did have a forceful personality; a fact that was pointed out to the author by other members of the cockpit and cabin crews. It is not unheard of for crew members to be intimidated by others who have more experience or seniority or who are more dynamic. The collision of the two Boeing 747s on the ground in Tenerife in 1977 is but one example of this. It has been reported that the First Officer of the KLM aircraft failed to act in the way he knew to be correct because the Captain, Jacob Louis Veldhuyzen van Zanten, was the airline's most senior captain and he was in awe of him.

When the fire broke out as Whisky Echo left the ground, the crew must have been reminded of the fire that it had suffered the previous November. As the accident report pointed out:

> ...latent fears in the minds of the crew that the fire might not be controllable were heightened by the knowledge of a recent accident to a Boeing 707 aircraft at Honolulu – involving this aircraft – when the disintegration of a turbine wheel during take-off punctured a fuel tank. It is unlikely that the resulting fire in that case could have been put out in the air.

This must have terrified them all. The engine part which failed, causing the accident in Honolulu, was different from that onboard the aircraft on 8 April and in Honolulu Whisky Echo was still on the ground when it caught fire, so was able to stop immediately and evacuate the passengers and crew at once. The accident in April put them all in a much worse position as the fire did not start until they were airborne and, because of the conditions on the ground, their landing options were extremely limited. They had just taken off from what was, at that time, the busiest airport in Europe and one of the busiest in the world. The ground surrounding the airfield was densely populated and there was no alternative space in which a Boeing 707 could land, so they knew they had no choice but to return to Heathrow. When ATCO John Davis in the control tower cleared the aircraft to land on runway 05R they also knew that it would be a difficult approach and landing.

The fire on the port wing and in the No. 2 engine took hold very quickly and burned with such ferocity that they must have believed it was only a matter of minutes before the fuel tanks exploded, killing them all and possibly countless people on the ground. The Captain also knew, from the aircraft's load sheet, that one of the items of cargo in the hold was radioactive, which was dangerous in itself and more so in the event of an accident. They were all under extreme pressure to make sure that every one of their actions had a positive result and they had hardly any time at all to do everything that was necessary.

When one considers the ferocity of the fire and the fact that the flight, from the take-off on runway 28L to the superb landing on runway 05R, took exactly three minutes and thirty-two seconds – less time than it takes to boil an egg – the survival of 121 of the 126 people on board is nothing short of a miracle.

Chapter 9

A Lonely and Courageous Action

Soon after the investigations into the cause of the crash had begun many people had started to think about how the crew of Whisky Echo could have their efficiency and bravery rewarded.

Her Majesty the Queen's message to Cliff Taylor had been passed on to him but, apart from the many articles in the national newspapers in the days following the accident suggesting that awards would be appropriate, no mention of any official recognition, based on eyewitness accounts, was noted until 19 April.

Eleven days after the accident Mr H.J. Judd, the technical assistant to Mr D. Doran, the occupational health engineer at the ACJMS, sent a report to the BOAC deputy personnel manager, Mr K. Daly, giving details of what Brian and Shirley Cooper had said about Jane Harrison:

> I assisted in collecting and looking after a number of the passengers who had been brought to the ACJMS Medical Unit at BEA West and, after treatment, those not requiring hospitalisation were made comfortable in the nurses' rest room in this unit. Tea was distributed to the passengers and I encouraged conversation, including accounts of the accident to relieve tension and shock. In the course of these conversations, Mr. Cooper expressed the greatest admiration for Miss Harrison's bravery, claiming that he saw flames licking around her and in spite of this she continued to assist passengers to leave the aircraft. Further expressions of admiration were voiced by some of the other survivors.
>
> I also spoke to the B.A.A. Fire Officer who entered the

burned out aircraft and saw the bodies of the victims: according to this officer the bodies were huddled together at the rear port exit. One of the victims was a very large person, and in the opinion of this officer, Miss Harrison returned to assist this passenger, when the final explosion occurred overwhelming all who remained behind.

I trust that these few observations are of help to you.

The report was stamped as having been received on 22 April and the following day Conservative MP for Kingston-upon-Thames, John Boyd-Carpenter, wrote to the President of the Board of Trade, Anthony Crosland. In his letter he said:

I wonder if you will allow me as one who at one time was responsible for Civil Aviation,[1] to put to you a suggestion which has probably also in any event occurred to you.

All the accounts of the accident to the BOAC Boeing at London Airport the other day indicate that the stewardess who was killed behaved with very great courage and self-sacrifice. She appears to have remained at her post, getting the passengers out until it was too late to save herself, and indeed according to some accounts actually went back into the cabin for this purpose. Although I know nothing of the girl and her family I am quite sure that it would be a great consolation to them if Her Majesty were to confer some appropriate posthumous award on her, and I am quite sure it would be very much appreciated by the cabin staff of our airlines.

I hope you will feel able to consider this, and if you have already in fact decided to act accordingly, please forgive me.

By now it was becoming obvious to BOAC that Jane Harrison, before losing her life on 8 April, had been rather more brave than they had, at first, believed.

On 24 April a Mr Brown of the Board of Trade had raised the question of a possible award for Jane. This led Group Captain J.B. Veal, Director General at the Civil Aviation Department of the Board of Trade, to write in a minute of 29 April:

The evidence available about the actions of the stewardess, Miss Harrison, is limited to what has been given by Steward Taylor and Stewardess Suares.

According to Steward Taylor, prior to the landing Stewardess Harrison was near to tears and he instructed her to strap herself into a jump seat which is adjacent to the rear main door. As soon as the aircraft came to a halt the Steward opened the rear galley door and operated the chute. At this point he remembers that Miss Harrison was behind him. When the chute was out she was no longer there. Stewardess Suares who was at the forward end of the aircraft looked towards the rear of the aircraft after landing and saw Stewardess Harrison standing in the aisle at approximately seat row 23, i.e. six rows from the rear of the aircraft.

Steward Taylor left the aircraft by the chute from the rear galley door as soon as the chute had deployed in order to reposition it and displace it from the flames which were spreading from the left-hand side of the aircraft. Subsequently five other people escaped by this chute before it became engulfed in flames. There is no evidence that Stewardess Harrison left by this chute and returned to the aircraft, nor would it have been practicable for her to return.

It appears that Stewardess Harrison was upset before the landing but after the landing it is believed that she did her job of assisting the passengers and that she was overcome by smoke.

Before he finished dictating this minute, Group Captain Veal had received information about the report written by Mr Judd and added to the minute:

This statement, a copy of which is being sent to me, apparently records laudatory remarks made by two of the passengers, Mr. and Mrs. Cooper, about the conduct of Stewardess Harrison and suggests a considerable degree of bravery and self-sacrifice on her part. BOAC are seeking statements from Mr. and Mrs. Cooper. In the circumstances there may well be reason to consider a posthumous award for Stewardess Harrison.

While BOAC waited for a response to their request for more details from Brian and Shirley Cooper who, with their two sons were, by this time, on board a ship taking them out to the Western Australian port of Fremantle, their deputy chairman, Keith Granville, had written to Anthony Crosland himself. Curiously although his letter, like that of John Boyd-Carpenter, was on the subject of awards, Granville completely ignored the part that Jane Harrison had played in saving passengers from flight BA 712. His letter, which he said he was writing on behalf of the chairman and board of BOAC, concentrated entirely on inviting the president of the Board of Trade to favourably consider a request for the award of George Medals to be presented to Captain Cliff Taylor and to Chief Steward Neville Davis-Gordon:

> ...in recognition of their action and behaviour on the occasion of the accident at London Airport to aircraft G-ARWE on 8 April 1968.

On the same day that he made this request, 8 May, Keith Granville also wrote to Secretary of State at the Board of Trade, John Mallalieu, who had accompanied both him and Sir Giles Guthrie when they visited the scene of the accident to Whisky Echo on 8 April. In this, much less formal note, he said:

> I enclose a formal letter which in Giles Guthrie's absence abroad I have written to the President of the Board of Trade. I am sending it through you because of the conversation which you and I had one evening in London when you asked that you should be kept in touch with this matter.
>
> I hope very much that the Board of Trade will support these recommendations for George Medals and advise us fully if by any chance we have not completed the citations adequately, or have fallen short in any way in our method of presentation. As I said to you when we last discussed this we think it very important indeed that the awards to be given to the Captain and Chief Steward should be made not later than the Birthday Honours list this year, which leaves awfully little time.

You will also be interested to know that on 24 May the BOAC Board will present Certificates of Commendation to the Captain, the technical staff and the cabin staff involved in the accident. We still have some problems with the citation for our own Certificate of Commendation for the Engineer Officer but I am hoping that these will be cleared in time for him to be included amongst those receiving the presentations.

When the day of the BOAC presentation came and the crew turned up for the ceremony, Andrew McCarthy recalled being upset at the absence of Flight Engineer Thomas Hicks. He suggested to Neville Davis-Gordon that none of them should accept the award if the Flight Engineer was going to be excluded. This conversation was overheard by one of the BOAC officials who was at pains to inform the two stewards that Thomas Hicks had, indeed, been given a Certificate of Commendation, but because it had been decided that he qualified for one rather later than the rest of the crew, due to the ongoing enquiry, his award had been made separately. Andrew was never sure whether Thomas Hicks did get the award as described by the official or whether it was an off the cuff excuse to avoid a scene at the presentation.

As well as the Certificates of Commendation each crew member had also been awarded an extra two weeks' holiday and confirmed air tickets to anywhere within the Sterling currency area for a fully paid holiday for themselves and a family member. John Hutchinson and his wife, Sue, went to Trinidad while Andrew McCarthy and his wife, Christina, chose Barbados, which was also the destination of Rosalind Unwin and her mother, where they stayed at the Coral Beech hotel.

Two days after Keith Granville had suggested to Anthony Crosland that the Captain and Chief Steward should be given awards, the British Airlines Stewards and Stewardesses Association of the Transport and General Workers Union sent a letter to Prime Minister Harold Wilson, in which they said:

At a full meeting of the British Airlines Stewards and

Stewardesses Association B.O.A.C. Branch 1/1261 on the 7th May 1968, a motion was proposed and carried unanimously, recommending,

"That our colleagues on the crew of the BA 712 which caught fire immediately after take-off from Heathrow Airport on the 8th April 1968, should be awarded an Official Decoration for their commendable action during the incident."

All of us in B.O.A.C. are very proud of the way in which the entire crew helped to avert, what could have been a major disaster, and we should like to show our appreciation by requesting some form of official recognition.

The letter was signed by P.R. Milani, the branch secretary and D.E. Brackley, branch chairman.

After Sir Giles Guthrie returned from his trip abroad he wrote to Anthony Crosland himself, inviting him to support the BOAC Board's 'very strong recommendation' that a posthumous award of the George Medal should be made to Jane Harrison and received the following reply, dated 29 May:

I am a writing to thank you for your letter of 15th May, and enclosure, about an award for Stewardess Barbara Harrison, who lost her life in the Boeing accident.

I am also acknowledging the letter of 8th May, and enclosure, which Keith Granville sent on behalf of yourself and the Board of BOAC, recommending awards for Captain Taylor and Chief Steward Davis-Gordon.

As you know, evidence is still being collected about the accident and it will be some months before the inquiry is completed. However, I assure you that the question of awards to the crew is something I myself have been considering. Your recommendations are a helpful contribution to this difficult question.

**

Six days after arriving in Western Australia, Brian and Shirley Cooper replied to a letter they had received from a Miss Cook at BOAC. Considering what they and their two boys had been through, it says much for the young couple that they set aside their own grief and replied promptly to the letter, giving details of what had happened to them and what they thought about what Jane Harrison had done. The handwritten letter told Miss Cook that they had had a good trip out to Australia and had spent a few days with Brian Cooper's sister who lived there, before moving to Point Walter[2] for what they hoped would be a few days or, perhaps weeks, until they could buy their own house and settle down.

They then said that they wanted to give their story of:

...the Stewardess Barbara Harrison, who died in the air crash Whisky Echo.

Miss Barbara Harrison was a very brave and courageous young lady. The last I saw of her was desperately trying to throw and encourage other passengers to jump from the plane. She threw me out through the side of the plane, smoke and flames licking around her face. I had only landed but a few moments when my wife threw my son and then jumped herself. As I got them to safety, I turned to go back to the plane, and I saw Barbara reappear, with another passenger, still with flames and explosions all around her, then complete blackness as she disappeared once more inside of the plane. That was the last my wife and myself ever saw of her, then we were taken away.

The letter was signed by Brian Cooper and a postscript added:

If this story is going to help you in any way in connection with Barbara Harrison, we have gladly given it, in our own words, how we saw it. Also if it wasn't for her quick action, no one would have survived, or at least not so many. We thank her although she is no longer with us.

When the letter was received in England copies were sent to various people within BOAC one of whom, the General Manager Flight Operations, Mr T. Nisbet, forwarded a copy to Group Captain Veal at the Board of Trade.

Meanwhile Her Majesty the Queen had been taking a personal interest in the awards to be made to the crew. In particular she was concerned with Captain Taylor's award and had brought up the subject at least twice. This led Michael Halls, principal private secretary to Prime Minister Harold Wilson, to write to Anthony Crosland in June 1968:

At the time of the submission of the recent Birthday List, The Queen enquired about the position of Captain Taylor and She was reminded that when She made her earlier enquiries we had pointed out that it was the practice in cases of this kind to await the result of the enquiry.

I should therefore be grateful if the consideration of the appropriate recognition for Captain Taylor can be arranged that if the President recommends an award, we can, if it seems appropriate and sensible at the time, announce it more or less simultaneously with the result of the enquiry.

Having made the point that awards were usually announced with the results of the enquiry, nothing of any significance happened during the rest of 1968. However, when the results of the enquiry were completed in April 1969, one year after the tragedy, the subject of the awards was resurrected and more letters went back and forth between the Prime Minister's private secretary, the Board of Trade and Stuart Milner-Barry, the civil servant who administered the British honours system. By May 1969 Milner-Barry, who had been both an England chess player and one of the leading code breakers at Bletchley Park during the Second World War, had collected a large amount of information about the actions of the various nominees for the awards, including the report of the enquiry, and had sent a letter to the Board of Trade in which he said:

We have looked carefully at the report here, and in the light of it I would agree with the Board of Trade view that the outstanding people to recommend for an honour are the Chief Steward and Miss Harrison. In all the circumstances it does seem difficult to recommend Captain Taylor or any of the flight crew. ...The Chief Steward who directed the operations behaved with coolness and efficiency. Miss Harrison was in the rear of the aircraft, which was the first part of the fuselage to be overwhelmed by the fire, and it appears that when the escape chute failed she threw some of the passengers out of the aircraft and encouraged others to jump. Apparently, she made no attempt to escape herself but remained behind with four passengers and with them died in the fire.

...If there is sufficient evidence to confirm what is said in the letter from Mr. Cooper...there would in my view be a good case for putting forward a recommendation for the award of a posthumous George Cross for Miss Harrison.

By the middle of June Prime Minister Harold Wilson's private secretary, Michael Halls, had contacted the Board of Trade asking if the president, Anthony Crosland, would let him know what he felt about the recommendations for the award of a George Cross to Jane Harrison and a British Empire Medal for Gallantry to Neville Davis-Gordon, but nothing for Captain Cliff Taylor. He also disclosed that Wilson wondered if it might be advisable to delay the decision until after the report of the enquiry had been published on 8 August so that the public mood could be properly assessed.

Anthony Crosland sent a confidential memo direct to Harold Wilson in Downing Street on 26 June, giving details of why it was felt that the two cabin crew members should receive awards but the cockpit crew should not. He believed that the report and the announcement of the awards should be made simultaneously and disclosed that:

After they had seen a copy of the Report, in confidence, the Chairman and the Managing Director of BOAC withdrew the recommendation which they had earlier submitted to me for an award for the captain.

After careful consideration of all the information available to me I do not think it would be appropriate to make any recommendation for an award to Captain Taylor. I believe that when the full circumstances of the accident are known, the aviation industry as a whole will accept that this decision is just.

Despite this assertion, there were those who thought that Whisky Echo's Captain did deserve recognition and Cliff Taylor was awarded the British Air Line Pilots Association Gold Medal for his expertise in bringing the aircraft back to Heathrow. Anthony Crosland approved the awards recommended by Stuart Milner-Barry for Neville Davis-Gordon and Jane Harrison, of whom he said:

> I also feel strongly that Miss Harrison's lonely and coura-geous action in that part of the aircraft first to be affected by heat and smoke when the integrity of the cabin was breached by an explosion should be recognised. From the evidence available, it is known that without thought for her own safety she returned time and again to the cabin door to push out a passenger before returning for another, until she went back into the aircraft and failed to reappear. I believe that this devotion to duty, in the highest traditions of her calling, is worthy of recognition by the posthumous award of the George Cross.

Michael Halls replied to the Board of Trade, on behalf of Harold Wilson, on the last day of July 1969:

> The Prime Minister has read your letter and has noted the President's further advice against any award to Captain Taylor – advice which the Prime Minister accepts. The Prime Minister has also noted that the President is confident that he can deal effectively with possible criticisms which may be made at the time about the decision not to recognise Captain Taylor.
>
> The Prime Minister has accordingly made his submission to The Queen recommending the award posthumously of the George Cross to Miss Barbara Harrison and the award of the B.E.M. for Gallantry to Mr. N.C. Davies-Gordon. [sic] The Queen is also being informed of the reasons why Captain Taylor is not being recognised.

Sadly for Cliff Taylor, although he had done nothing wrong and despite his brilliant landing the year before, he would be held accountable for the errors within the cockpit, simply because he was the aircraft's commander at the time of the accident.

***

In view of the amount of time it eventually took to decide which awards were to be given and to whom, it was interesting that in May 1968 Keith Granville should have been pushing for awards for the Captain and Chief Steward to be made: '...not later than the Birthday Honours list this year, which leaves awfully little time'. The letter asking for this was written only a month after the accident and it does seem strange that he was in such a rush to get the awards approved. The Birthday Honours are usually announced sometime in mid June; in this case only a month after Granville's letter. It is possible that the inordinate haste with which he acted was because he knew that if the awards were delayed until the results of the official enquiry were published, it was unlikely that the Captain would be honoured at all.

In the same month that Granville had written to Anthony Crosland, the results of BOAC's own investigation were published internally. The airline's Chief Inspector of Accidents was able to complete his enquiries much quicker than the Board of Trade investigators because the airline was just looking at its own part in the incident and did not, therefore, devote the large amount of time and effort that the Board of Trade did to the emergency services.

The following year, just before the official report was published, BOAC was sent its copy. Having read it, it was concluded by an unnamed person in the airline that:

> Its findings are similar to those of BOAC's Chief Inspector of Accidents whose report was circulated to Management in May 1968, but it additionally questions the efficiency and effectiveness of the airport fire service.
>
> Newspapers may well highlight this criticism of the fire service but it would be unreasonable to expect, because of this, that the Report's comments on BOAC emergency drills and on the conduct of the crew will be ignored.

The plain fact is that the fire service would not have been needed – and five lives would not have been lost – had no mistakes been made on the flight deck.[3]

The document, in which this astonishingly frank and simplistic opinion is given, runs to fourteen pages and, although unsigned, appears to have been written by a senior official within the airline, as it gives answers that would be acceptable to BOAC should questions be asked by journalists regarding the results of the official enquiry. The paragraph which follows says:

The image of BOAC's technical crews, and that of BOAC itself, will probably be tarnished. The degree to which this happens may depend in part on how Press Officers deal with inquiries and 'field' the more awkward questions.

One of the awkward situations envisaged by the writer of this document was about the crew responsibilities:

We will be asked about the crew and the Captain's responsibilities. It may be suggested that because he was the commander, Captain Taylor was responsible for what happened. If we are asked does BOAC hold Captain Taylor responsible we should say: 'No – Captain Taylor had correctly delegated certain duties to other members of his crew and had a right to expect them to be carried out. He had to make an immediate and difficult emergency landing and all his attentions would have been occupied with this.

...A lengthy report, discussing in academic and abstract terms what must have been a horrifying experience, does not convey the sense of urgency and emergency the crew must have felt.

We may be asked why, in fact, the crew, particularly the EO, FO and Check Captain are still flying – some of the newspapers know that they were reprimanded.

Reprimands – and who they are given to – are an internal matter. We shouldn't discuss them.

The document also disclosed that, contrary to what had been told to Andrew McCarthy and Neville Davis-Gordon:

...all members of the technical crew, except the EO, were given commendations by the Board of BOAC... .

In the week before the publication of the enquiry report, while BOAC was refining its damage limitation strategy, letters went out to Neville Davis-Gordon and to Jane's father, Alan Harrison, announcing the awards. The news was made public three days later, 8 August 1969, in a supplement to *The London Gazette*. Kay Golightly, Jane's friend, vividly remembered hearing the news that day; it was her twenty-fifth birthday.

Three days after the announcement Captain Cliff Taylor wrote to Alan Harrison saying:

Please excuse me for not writing to you prior to this. The loss of your daughter Jane, must have been a great loss to you. Words written or spoken at such times do not seem to help much. Believe me my sympathy was, and still is, a very real thing.

I am delighted that her great sacrifice has now been officially recognised, by the award of the George Cross. You must be a very proud man. Be assured that we who fly are also very proud of your daughter.

On 4 September Alan Harrison was the guest of honour at a lunch at the RAF club given by Sir John Smyth VC and other members of the Victoria Cross and George Cross Association.

Although his name had not appeared in the large amount of correspondence relating to the accident to Whisky Echo and the awards to the crew, one more person who had been involved in the incident also received an honour. This award had not been the subject of any dispute and, on 5 May 1969, Air Traffic Control Officer John Davis received a letter from No. 10 Downing Street informing him that he was to be awarded a well deserved MBE.[4]

Alan Harrison went to the investiture at Buckingham Palace on

Wednesday 29 October to accept the George Cross on behalf of his daughter. Jane's sister, Sue, could have gone to London with her father but she had recently given birth to her first child and so remained in Yorkshire and Alan was accompanied by Jane's stewardess friend, Susan Perry.

Chief Steward Neville Davis-Gordon went to Buckingham Palace to receive his British Empire Medal with his wife, Diddy, and daughter, Carole, and Air Traffic Control Officer John Davis attended with his wife, Jaqi, and their children Linda and Andrew. While presenting Neville Davis-Gordon with his BEM, the Queen told him that Prince Philip had been watching Whisky Echo as it made its terrifying last flight into Heathrow.

All three awards – the George Cross, BEM for Gallantry and the MBE – were richly deserved, but what of the rest of the people involved in the accident to Whisky Echo? When he learned of his award, Neville Davis-Gordon said:

> I am very pleased to have got the BEM, but I feel I owe the award to my cabin staff and their teamwork, and I shall accept it on their behalf.

In a statement, BOAC's deputy chairman and managing director, Keith Granville, declared:

> We in BOAC will always remember the heroism and bravery of Miss Harrison and Mr Davis-Gordon.
> They did their duty magnificently and we are very proud to be associated with them.

What no one from BOAC mentioned was that the five men in the cockpit on that fateful day had also played their part in saving so many people from the fire. Mistakes may have been made – some would say this was perfectly understandable given the ferocity of the fire, the loss of an engine and the very short time between take-off and landing – but without their skill in bringing the aircraft back home and safely landing it, no one would have been saved and there might have been many more deaths on the ground as well. It should be remembered that any take-off brings with it numerous tasks and checks for the men in the cockpit to complete and, with the failure of the No. 5 low pressure compressor wheel and the resulting fire, their work was made almost impossible. They had 212 seconds from take-off to landing to go through all these checks, turn the aircraft, make a difficult approach to a runway that was not as well equipped as those usually used and then land, knowing that they might not have enough time to get back onto the ground safely and that, even if they did make it, there was a fierce fire burning on the wing, they had a lot of fuel onboard and there were 115 passengers and a total of eleven crew who would all have to get off very quickly if they were to survive.

The aviation industry may have understood from a purely technical point of view why the cockpit crew were not recommended for awards – mistakes had been made – but, knowing what those men went through during those 212 seconds, and appreciating that their actions in bringing back the crippled aircraft gave the 115 passengers on board a chance, however small, to live, many of them felt that justice had not been served at all.

Chapter 10

Then and Now

The days following the accident had been filled with activity; those injured in the accident recovered in hospital, other survivors made alternative travel arrangements, companies with cargo on board Whisky Echo started to make claims for compensation, as did individuals whose letters had been destroyed in the fire – surprisingly many appeared to contain postal orders – and BOAC cleared away the wreckage, bought a replacement 707 and got back to the business of running an airline.

Australian Diane Johnson, who was living in London and had written to her mother in Sydney, discovered that her letter had been on board Whisky Echo. Interviewed on an Australian television programme on 5 September 2005 she recalled how the remains of her letter had arrived:

> ...it's rather quaint what happened when it got to Sydney. In those days it was the Postmaster General's Department. And the wording's quite quaint. It did arrive on 3 May, which is a month later, and it says, 'Dear Madam, the attached article was salvaged from the aircraft which crashed at London Heathrow airport on 8 April 1968. Please accept my apologies for the inconvenience which you have experienced as a result of this incident.'

BOAC engineer Doug Cotterell's sons, David and Allen, received the letter their grandmother had written to them even later. In a note, sent on behalf of the Postmaster-General of Singapore and dated 17 May, they were told:

I forward herewith an airmail letter which has been received from the British Post Office in a batch of correspondence salvaged from the ill-fated BOAC aircraft which crashed at London Airport on 8 April, 1968.

I am sorry for the damage caused to the letter.

Having survived the ordeal on Whisky Echo, Eric Blower had returned to his home in Leeds by train. Although his company, IAL, had, at first, insisted that he had to work his three months' probationary period before his wife and daughter would be eligible to join him in Australia, they relented because of what he had been through and, on 22 April, Eric's wife, Rita, and their daughter, Nicola, joined him on the flight to their new home in Perth. They had been booked on the same flight – BA 712 – as Eric had two weeks before:

Same time, same place, same number! I knew it was now or never. Had I put it off any longer I would never have gone. The Company arranged an appointment to see the BOAC doctor at Heathrow prior to the flight. Thank heaven for Valium (I didn't need an aeroplane, I had my own wings!) We did actually fly from Leeds to Heathrow that morning but don't ask me how! Probably hadn't properly sobered up from the night before!

We arrived in Perth all in one piece on the 24th and lived and worked there for 4+ years. It was lovely. We actually sailed back home from Fremantle to the UK in August 1972. (Seven weeks of heaven.)

I spent the rest of my working life travelling with IAL (flying not a problem). Loved every minute of it. Nightmares? Yes, for about 3 years after the accident then gladly they faded away.

Sadly Rita Blower died of cancer in 1981. After Eric retired from IAL he met Denise, who became his wife in 1998. His daughter Nicola now lives in the Middle East.

Canon and Mrs Henn, after their interview with the *West Australian* newspaper, were reunited with their son Basil and met their granddaughter, Susan, for the first time. The couple went on to Bunbury where the Canon eventually became Archdeacon Emeritus of the Diocese of Bunbury. He died in 1987 at the age of eighty. Mrs Henn survived him and, just after the fortieth anniversary of her ordeal on board Whisky Echo, will celebrate her 100th birthday.

Having informed friends and relatives via the television news that he was safe, Richard Hamond was given an extra two weeks to take up his new job in Australia and so went back to Norfolk the day after the accident. That evening he went to his local pub where his fishermen friends informed him that they had not been worried about him at all as they knew it would take more than an air crash to get rid of him! When the two extra weeks had passed the marine biologist once more boarded an aircraft bound for Sydney where he lived and worked for four years. He then took up a position at the university in Melbourne and stayed for another thirteen years, described by him as the best years of his life, before returning to his native Norfolk where he still lives in the house in which he grew up.

Mark Wynter married his fiancée, Janeece, as planned on Friday 19 April. Three days later he was at the Chevron Hotel in St Kilda Road, Melbourne to fulfil his cabaret engagement. The events of 8 April seem to have been pushed to the back of his mind and the review in the Melbourne newspaper*The Herald* the next day was full of praise for the performance. Headlined 'It's a cool and adult Wynter' the article went on to say that:

> In an age of built-in obsolescence, Mark Wynter is a rare showbiz character. A pop idol who has survived frenetic teenage fan-dom to become a cool, adult nightclub singer.
> ...In fact he approaches his songs rather like Frank Sinatra.

In a bizarre coincidence, on the same page of the newspaper was a short article about a South African Airways Boeing 707 bound for London from Johannesburg which had crashed soon after take-off with 128 passengers and crew on board. Unlike Whisky Echo, two weeks before, 122 people died in this accident. It really emphasized just how lucky Mark, and the other survivors, had been.

When the cabaret engagement finished in May, Mark and

Janeece took their delayed honeymoon. They visited Ischia and Rome but before they had even left Australia on the honeymoon trip there was more aviation related drama for the young singer. The flight to Italy went via Perth and soon after the aircraft left the ground heading for Singapore they felt it make a turn and come back in towards the airport. This time there was no fire but the airline had received a bomb threat and so the aircraft returned to Perth for an emergency landing. It was later that Mark and his wife discovered that the likely reason for the threat – a hoax – was that the Governor General of New South Wales was on board.

Sadly the Wynters' marriage did not last, but Mark married for a second time and now has two sons and a daughter and a very successful acting career. He feels that he was extremely lucky to have survived the Whisky Echo tragedy.

John Molineaux, his wife, Lilian and children Irene and John decided that they didn't want to fly to Australia after all and so took up the Australian migration department's offer of a sea passage and arrived in Perth by boat. John worked for EBM Insurance Brokers for over 10 years before retiring to Cairns in Queensland in 1987.[1]

When Donald Hay and his wife, Patricia, decided that they would like to emigrate, the only one of their five children who didn't want to go was fourteen year old Trevor. Now he is glad that he did as he says that he 'fell on his feet'. His brother and sisters are scattered across the country now. Diane, who was twelve at the time of the accident, married but is now divorced and still lives in Perth. Cheryl, the younger of the twins, is also still living in Perth. Lorraine, the other twin, joined the Australian Army and served in Timor during the troubles there. She now lives in Brisbane but, sadly, has multiple sclerosis. Kevin moved to New South Wales where he has a horse breeding ranch in Goulburn.

When Trevor and his family escaped from the burning aircraft they were looked after by a BOAC ground hostess. Nearly forty years later Trevor still keeps in touch with the lady he affectionately refers to as 'Aunty Sandi'. At the time of the accident he collected all the press cuttings he could find and kept them in a folder. One day Kevin was looking for a folder and the only one he could find was the one containing Trevor's press cuttings. Kevin didn't stop to check whether or not his brother would mind if he took it, he simply removed the collection – the record of what the entire family had lived through – and threw it away.

After he left school Trevor joined the Royal Australian Navy and served for twenty years before spending the next twelve years as a house husband. He then rejoined the Navy and is due to retire at the end of 2007. He has a son and a daughter.

Five years after the accident Trevor made an amazing discovery:

> Richard Hamond and I almost got together a few years after the crash – although he doesn't know it. As I mentioned, I joined the Royal Australian Navy and in 1973 went to the Naval College at Jervis Bay. I was surprised one day when one of our instructors started talking about a doctor coming to the college the previous year to lecture on oceanography, but who (apparently) showed a lot of photos about a plane crash from the inside. As I listened it became obvious that it was 'my' plane crash and then it was the instructor's turn to be surprised when I told him that I was seated next to the doctor. The world is incredibly small.

Trevor is still a Southampton football supporter and, when the team was building its new stadium at St Mary's, he bought one of the bricks which formed part of the new ground and has his name on it. Sadly he still doesn't have the team's autographs!

For Fred and Vera Pragnell and their children the move to Australia was a success and they remain in Perth. With the children now grown up and leading their own lives, Fred, known to his friends as Freddo, and Vera have been able to spend more time on their love of musical theatre. They both appeared in a production of *Les Miserables* and, at the end of 2007, in a show called *Paris*, about Paris and Helen of Troy with music by Sir Elton John. Fred also builds sets for the stage and paints backdrops. He has a great sense of humour and is always busy. As he says:

...in my spare time I repair computers, all for love, so you can
imagine a lot of people love me...!

For the Cooper family the spectre of Whisky Echo was to haunt
them for many more years. The other immigrant families had
the excitement of a new country and a new life to help them
forget but Brian and Shirley had to learn to live without their
only daughter; Kevin and Andrew without their sister. It was
perhaps easier for Andrew who was so young when Jacky died
that his memory of her was hazy. For Kevin it was very difficult.
He and Jacky had been so close and he missed her a lot. His
parents both think that he never really got over her loss.

After they moved into the Point Walter hostel they became
friendly with the English family who were living in the next
door hut. Sue Palmer née Joyce remembered how she and her
sister used to play with the Cooper boys:

> I do remember them coming down to Golden Bay with us
> often. My sister and I had both learned to swim whilst still
> in UK and had all sorts of achievement certificates for it. I
> remember a time on the beach down there when we took our
> foam surf boards out with the two Cooper boys and all got
> caught in a rip. My sister and I had to pull them out as they
> couldn't swim at all. We hadn't known that at the time. That
> incident had a huge effect on me and I never went into the
> sea any deeper than my ankles until I met my husband 15
> years ago. He was an avid triathlete and helped me back
> into the sea again so that eventually I was able to compete in
> all three legs of the event instead of only two!

Two years after they arrived in Australia, Brian Cooper almost
decided to return to England as he was finding it difficult to
settle. However, they had found themselves a home and had
made friends and, as time passed, the family's lives did return
to normal and they were glad that they had stayed. After they
had been in Perth for a while, Brian and Shirley decided to have
another baby and a daughter they called Michelle was born.
Then, in 1985, their lives were torn apart again.

Kevin met a girl and got married. About six months after the wedding things were not going well and the couple split up. When the marriage ended in divorce, Kevin became very depressed. This, after the loss of his sister, was too much for him to bear and he committed suicide. After the funeral his ashes were brought back to England where they were buried in the same grave as Jacqueline.

Despite their lives having been touched by so much grief, Brian and Shirley Cooper have survived. Things did not turn out as they had planned and they have had more than their fair share of troubles but they have come through them all. They have their friends, their family which now also includes two grandchildren – Michelle's son and daughter – and their shared interest in the local soccer club. Most of all they have each other and, in March 2008, they will celebrate their golden wedding.

Seventeen months after the accident, on 17 September 1969, the inquest into the deaths of Jane Harrison, Jacqueline Cooper, Esther Cohen, Catherine Shearer and Mary Smith was held. The inquest verdict was 'Accidental Death' and it was stated that they had died of 'Asphyxia due to Inhalation of Fire Fumes'.

For some of the crew on board Whisky Echo, life continued but was never quite the same again. Cliff Taylor had been planning to retire but the fact that his life had been spared on that April day made him change his mind. He said that he felt he had to go on after that and so put his retirement plans on hold. Although he had spoken of perhaps going to live in Australia when he did eventually retire he remained in England, in the same house in which he had lived in 1968. He died in January 2006.

First Officer Francis Kirkland and Flight Engineer Thomas Hicks carried on flying for BOAC but both are now retired.

When a firm of printers in Letchworth, Hertfordshire, learned that Acting First Officer John Hutchinson had been on board Whisky Echo and that his logbook had been damaged in the fire, they offered to repair it for him. They returned the book, beautifully restored and refused to take any payment for the work that they had done. The entry in the logbook for 8 April 1968 simply reads:

FIRE NO. 2 ENGINE EX LHR.   SAFE LANDING 05R.
AIRCRAFT DESTROYED.

John continued to fly on Boeing 707s until February 1971 when
he transferred to the Boeing 747. In October 1975 he became a
VC10 captain, flying this aircraft for the next two years, after
which he spent nearly fifteen years as a Concorde pilot. In the
mid 1980s he was asked to do a piece for television for a show
about the Battle of Britain and did so from a Concorde flying at
6,000 feet. It was recognized that he was a natural broadcaster
and he has appeared in many programmes since about the
British Airways Concordes and the one belonging to Air France
which crashed in July 2000 in Paris.

Neville Davis-Gordon continued to fly as a chief steward and,
when he gave up flying, became a councillor in Bournemouth.
In 1993, shortly after undergoing a medical in which he was
declared fit, he suffered a heart attack at his home and died aged
sixty-four.

Andrew McCarthy also continued his flying career. In 1970 he
was posted for a time to New Zealand. Then, in 1971 back in
England, he became Chief Steward. He retired in 2001 and he
and his wife Christina are the proud grandparents of twin boys.

Stewardess Jennifer Suares was based in Delhi and after the
accident returned home but remained with BOAC. Passenger
Richard Hamond remembered seeing her in Sydney sometime
later and asked her if she would like to see the photos he had
taken of Whisky Echo but she preferred not to, letting the events
of 8 April remain in the past.[2]

When she returned to her home in Coventry, Rosalind Unwin
found herself being hailed a heroine. The term made her feel
uncomfortable as she has always maintained that she was
simply one of a team who worked together to help as many
people as possible escape. Despite this she was asked to appear
in a television interview which was filmed in her back garden as
her mother refused to let her go to the television studio. She
was also invited to a number of events including a ceremony at
Combe Abbey near to Coventry. She was made a 'Citizen of
Coventry' and, with steward Bryan Taylor, was invited to a

dinner given in their honour by Luton Town Football club, Luton having once been Bryan's home town.[3]

Rosalind worked as a BOAC stewardess for a total of seven years. When she left the airline her love of sport offered her another career path and she became a squash professional and then a yoga teacher. Now married to husband Nick she still teaches yoga and the couple both enjoy overseas travel.

Bryan Taylor's career with BOAC was not to last. He was very upset about the accident and felt that he was responsible for Jane Harrison's death because he had left her in the aircraft while he got out to straighten the emergency chute.[4] He had some time off work after the accident but when he came back to the airport he was rostered to work a flight with Andrew McCarthy again. Andrew remembers being in the first class section of the aircraft just prior to the departure time and hearing a passenger say, 'Are you not staying with us then?' He turned to find Bryan behind him, holding his coat and bag. Bryan said that he was sorry but he couldn't work the flight and got off the aircraft.

Sometime later Andrew discovered that Bryan had left the airline and had become a pub landlord. He went to visit him and, although Bryan seemed pleased to see him, he told him that he didn't want any more contact from anyone at BOAC.[5]

For air traffic controller, John Davis, life returned to normal. Then, on 6 September 1970, he was again involved in a terrifying situation. At that time the Popular Front for the Liberation of Palestine was at its most active, having conducted several aircraft hijacks. Palestinian Leila Khaled, who had been involved with the hijacking of a TWA aircraft to Damascus the year before (see Appendix 4) and Patrick Argüello, son of a Nicaraguan father and an American mother, boarded a New York bound 707, belonging to the Israeli national airline El Al, in Amsterdam, posing as a Honduran married couple. As the aircraft approached the United Kingdom the couple, armed with guns and grenades, demanded to be allowed into the cockpit but a fight ensued with the aircraft's security staff, during which one of the stewards and Leila Khaled were injured, and Patrick Argüello was killed. One of the hijackers had thrown a grenade into the cockpit with the pin removed but it proved to be faulty and didn't explode. The Israeli pilot made a call to London and was given clearance by John Davis to land on runway 28R which was closed for some hours while the British security forces dealt with the situation and eventually arrested Leila Khaled, taking her to Hillingdon hospital to have her wounds treated.

Happily this hijack was the last unpleasant incident that John Davis had to deal with and he ended his air traffic control career when he retired in 1997, having transferred to Gatwick airport from Heathrow.

Jane Harrison's father Alan moved back to Yorkshire after his daughter's death. In 1987 he decided to sell Jane's George Cross. Some newspaper reports said he was selling it as he needed the money for his own living expenses. This was simply not true and other reports gave the true reason. In an article in *The Observer* dated 4 October 1987 (coincidentally Alan Harrison's birthday) writer Peter Watson said:

> After much soul-searching, Mr Harrison has decided there is no point in keeping a medal which will eventually be inherited by someone who never knew his daughter. Instead he will sell it and give the money to the children of his other daughter.
>
> They never knew Jane either, and Mr Harrison's unsentimental reaction is likely to shock some people. But he says: 'The honour is in the award, not the medal itself.'

The medal was included in a sale of other medals at Sotheby's on 29 October 1987, eighteen years to the day after it had been presented to Alan Harrison at Buckingham Palace. It was listed in the catalogue as:

THE EXCESSIVELY RARE POSTHUMOUS GEORGE CROSS, awarded to **Miss Barbara Jane Harrison, 8 August 1969 [Stewardess, B.O.A.C.]**, *on Ladies' riband bow and in case of issue, extremely fine* [**One of only four direct awards of the G.C. to women – this one being unique for the post war period**]

The citation which had appeared in *The London Gazette* on 8 August 1969 was also presented, along with a brief description of the accident taken from the official report, a copy of which was sold with the medal.

There had been fears that the medal would go to a foreign bidder and that the unique award would leave the country but this did not happen. As David Erskine-Hill of Sotheby's said:

> Its associations are so British that it would be nice to think it will appeal strongly to a British collector – or even to the newly-privatised British Airways.

When the hammer fell at the end of the auction and the medal was sold for £9,000, its buyer was, indeed, British Airways. The medal is now kept safely in a vault but a replica is displayed in the British Airways museum beside a photo of the girl who brought such honour to the airline.

Alan Harrison lived for twenty-eight more years after his daughter's untimely death and died in 1996, aged eighty-five. It seems that he was right to sell the medal as it is now at Heathrow airport, the place where Jane died, and remains a permanent reminder of her sacrifice. Her niece and nephew, Helen and Adrian, have also benefited, each having had money to help with their education. They made good use of it and both went on to gain university degrees. Although they never knew their brave aunt, they are both extremely proud of her.

Sue Buck, Jane's sister, and her husband Vic, now grandparents to Helen's children, have remained in Yorkshire where they have a lovely home with a beautiful garden in which Sue likes to work. A tall, elegant, quietly spoken lady, Sue speaks of her sister with humour, affection and pride but also with regret for what might have been. It has been hard for her to relive the events of forty years ago but she has done so, with grace and patience, for her sister.

Jane's friends have never forgotten the feisty, fun-loving girl they met at school either and, despite the passing of the years, she remains close to their hearts.

The three remaining members of the little gang of four from

Scarborough Girls High school no longer live close to each other. Kay is the only one to still live in the area in which she grew up. Margaret, who moved to Rome to work with the United Nations, still lives there with her husband and family. Sheila and her husband John moved to Australia in 1978. Their children have grown up and Sheila is now a grandmother. In a letter to the author in which she included a photo of herself and her family, Sheila wrote:

Me, now 63 (old aged pensioner!). How we have all changed!! How would Jane have aged??

It is sad to think of everything that Jane lost by her heroic act forty years ago – the chance of a life with a husband, children of her own, family and friends, her career – the things that her friends have had while she remains in their minds, and in the minds of all who knew her, a twenty-two year old girl who had everything to live for but who gave it all up for the sake of others.

Chapter 11

The Legacy of Jane Harrison

The death of any young person is a tragedy, however it occurs. When that person has died in an effort to save others there is, inevitably, great interest in the event and a desire in many people to do something to honour the sacrifice and so it was with Jane Harrison.

At the beginning of October 1969 Jane's father received a letter from Essex based aviation writer, Leslie Hunt. He was planning to write a book about George Cross holders who had been awarded their medals in aviation related incidents and had contacted BOAC for information about Jane. The airline had supplied a photo and had given Mr Hunt Alan Harrison's address, so he wrote asking for information, about Jane's early life and her interest in aviation, for his book. He enclosed with the letter a leaflet about muscular dystrophy saying that he donated the profits of his books to research into this disease and to aircraft preservation charities. By the end of October Alan Harrison had replied to the letter and had sent a donation for the Muscular Dystrophy Group research fund. It appears that he had also offered to help on an ongoing basis as Leslie Hunt's reply said:

> Your kind letter and generous donation came as a real inspiration to our small membership and we'd be very honoured to count you with us in the battle to find a cure for muscular dystrophy.
>
> ...It was most kind of you – and your daughter Susan – to take such trouble to help me and I've already taken the

liberty of getting air stewardesses at Southend Airport interested in some form of practical memorial to Jane – with your
permission.

The practical memorial that Mr Hunt had in mind was the
setting up of a fund in Jane's name which would provide much
needed equipment for a hospital to allow better diagnosis and
treatment for children with muscular dystrophy.

When he wrote again a few days later it was to tell Jane's
father how he proposed to launch an appeal and reassured him
that:

I'll not do anything pending your decision but am burning to
set this off so that Jane's glorious sacrifice is never forgotten
and in hopes that it might bring life to many boys and girls
who would otherwise die in their teens.

Alan Harrison agreed to Leslie Hunt's proposal and the Barbara
Jane Harrison, G.C., Memorial Fund was set up with the target
of raising £1,000[1] by October 1970.

An appeal was launched with advertisements in *Flight
International* and *BOAC News*, as well as various newspapers
and the cheques started to arrive at the Muscular Dystrophy
Group of Great Britain headquarters in Borough High Street,
south-east London.

Dorothy Morcam Taylor who, with her sister Helena, had
been a passenger on board Whisky Echo, wrote to Alan
Harrison in June 1970 to tell him that:

I have managed to do a little to help the Barbara Jane
Harrison G.C. Memorial Fund. I did succeed in getting from
the Wings Travel people the names and addresses of the
fellow members from [our] party and wrote to each one of
them. Most of them replied and said that they had sent a
contribution and were very glad to know of the fund.
Incidentally this brought us some interesting contacts and
we were able to compare notes from experiences. Last week
some friends of ours invited us to give a lecture with colour
transparencies of our last year's trip 'From Ceylon to the
Himalayas' in their home in Edgware. They got some

beautiful little hand drawn posters done 'in aid of the Barbara Jane Harrison G.C. Memorial Fund for Research into Muscular Dystrophy' and we raised £13 5s by it.[2] We wished it had been more but every little helps! Anyway I have kept the little posters in the hope that we might be able to give it again somewhere else before the fund closes, which I understand it does in August. Is that right?

When the fund finally closed in October it had raised nearly £1,500. The money had come from members of the public who were touched by the story of Jane's sacrifice, but also from passengers who had been on board Whisky Echo, airline crews and ground staff, including proceeds from a BOAC dance which raised £75, and pupils from Scarborough Girls High School. The money was used to purchase badly needed computer equipment. It was presented to the National Hospital in Queen Square, London, for use in its Muscular Dystrophy Group laboratories, on 23 October 1970. Attending the presentation were Professor John Cumings, who was in charge of the research project, Dr B.P. Hughes, one of the experts who would use the equipment, Leslie Hunt and Sir John Smyth, chairman of the Victoria Cross and George Cross Association. Soon afterwards a photo of Alan Harrison and Dr Hughes, with the computer equipment, appeared in the newspapers.

Before going to the National Hospital on 23 October to present the computer, Alan Harrison had been at Heathrow airport to attend the dedication of a plaque in Jane's memory at the Chapel of St George (see Appendix 2) and, following the service, BOAC had arranged for a car to take him to the hospital.

There were other memorials including one at St Lawrence's churchyard in Scalby, close to where Jane had lived as a child. The memorial is in the form of a round plaque, set into the wall by the entrance to the churchyard, giving details of Jane's bravery taken from the citation for her George Cross. Beneath it is a container which is always filled with fresh flowers, put there in memory of Jane by local residents Ken and Marie Gill.

Following Jane's funeral a headstone was place on her grave. After the award of the George Cross the inscription was amended to include this and it now reads:

HARRISON

LOVING THOUGHTS

OF

JANE

AGED 22 YEARS

B.O.A.C STEWARDESS WHO

DIED AT HEATHROW AIRPORT

ON 8TH APRIL 1968, TRYING TO

SAVE THE LIVES OF OTHERS FROM

THE BOEING 707 "WHISKY ECHO"

AWARDED THE "GEORGE CROSS"

In September 1969 the Old Girls Club from Scarborough Girls High School decided to donate something to the school in memory of Jane. A flower stand was suggested and commissioned. It was presented to the school in April 1970 and placed on the platform in the school hall in a ceremony attended by Jane's father.[3]

One of the girls who knew Jane at Scarborough Girls High was Vicky Ireland. They were close friends for a very short time before Vicky moved to Devon. When she left school Vicky trained as an actress and has specialized in children's theatre, acting, directing and writing. In a flyer about herself, produced for children, she answers the question 'Who is your best friend?' by saying:

> My first best friend at secondary school was Jane Harrison. She grew up to become an air hostess and was tragically killed trying to rescue a passenger from a plane crash. There is a window dedicated to her memory in the chapel at Heathrow. She was funny, loyal and always courageous. Then I moved schools and after that, I had a gang of best friends.

The window to which Vicky Ireland refers is likely to be the plaque in St George's Chapel at Heathrow but Jane's life is commemorated on a memorial window at Bradford City Hall along with those of twelve other local heroes and heroines. In 2000 Bradford City Council leader, Ian Greenwood said:

It's a shame that most Bradford people have never heard of these local heroes so I thought it was time their names were put on permanent record.

Their selfless acts of courage should never be forgotten. These brave men and women are a wonderful example to us and to future generations.

The memorial in Bradford is in the form of a gallery, with photos of the thirteen people and descriptions of their brave deeds, set in front of a window. It was unveiled at a ceremony on 27 March 2000 and the *Yorkshire Post* described how no one could trace any of Jane's relatives to invite to the unveiling. By July that year they had found her sister and brother-in-law and another article appeared in the *Yorkshire Post* with a photo showing the couple in front of the memorial and a quote from Vic Buck, who said:

Seeing the memorial you realize what a brave person she was and how devoted she was to her job.

To coincide with the sixtieth anniversary of the end of the Second World War the London Underground produced a series of posters highlighting some of the brave deeds that led to the awards of the country's highest honours – the Victoria and George Crosses. Each poster was dedicated to one person and described what he or she had done to receive the award. In the publicity which launched this memorial campaign, London Underground said that its slogan:

'Ordinary people, extraordinary deeds' reinforces the message that courage and altruism in the face of danger is a quality to which we can, each and every one of us, aspire.

Since no woman has ever been awarded a Victoria Cross, although it was not intended to be an honour for men alone, and only four women have ever been directly awarded a George Cross, the memorial campaign was, almost entirely, about men. However, in 2005, passengers travelling on the London Underground were also able to see a photo of Jane Harrison and read about what she had done in April 1968. This memorial, although not permanent, did at least introduce Jane and her story to many people who would not, otherwise, have heard of her.

The memorial that has made the name of Barbara Jane Harrison known across the world, however, is not a plaque or a monument or poster; it is a prize awarded to overseas students in the field of aviation medicine – a branch of occupational medicine concerned with human physiology and psychology in the alien conditions required for manned flight.

Dr Roger Green who, in 1968, was a newly-joined medical officer with the joint medical services of BEA and BOAC witnessed Whisky Echo landing in flames and described how the prize came into being:

> The Barbara Harrison Prize was established in her memory by the teaching staff of the Royal Air Force Institute of Aviation Medicine and is sponsored by British Airways, who first suggested the idea.
>
> In 1968 the Institute was tasked by the Royal College of Physicians of London with organising and running a six month full time course in Aviation Medicine, culminating in an examination for the award of a Diploma in Aviation Medicine. This subsequently became the responsibility of the Faculty of Occupational Medicine of the RCP, and has now devolved to the Department of Aviation Medicine at King's College at the University of London. ...The teaching for the course has always been a joint effort by the staff of the UK armed forces (mainly the RAF) and various representatives of civil aviation – both airlines and regulatory authorities in the UK.
>
> The course is attended by doctors from the armed services of the UK as well as many other countries, and from airlines from all over the world. The teaching is in English, of

course, and at the outset a prize was established (The Stewart Memorial Prize in memory of a former commandant of the Institute) for the outstanding student on the course. It was clear from the start that this would almost always be won by a student whose first language is English and it occurred to some of us who were involved in the teaching, but were airline people rather than Air Force, that an award for the best student whose first language is not English would be an appropriate way to recognise the international nature of the training. Quite how Barbara Jane's name was suggested for commemoration I am not sure but I know it was thought that the contribution of cabin crew to air safety was worthy of greater recognition.

It was Dr Green's former colleague, Dr Roy Maclaren, who initially suggested the name of the prize. He, too, knew that the role of cabin crew was vital to the wellbeing of passengers and that a prize in Jane's name would, therefore, be particularly appropriate. He also thought it important to recognize those students who sometimes struggled with having to take the course in what was, to them, a second language but who showed enormous enthusiasm for the task they had been set and spoke of:

...the unlikely link between an internationally respected group of doctors in specialist training and a young cabin crew member. The former began life prosaically in the same year as Barbara Jane surrendered hers heroically. We all need heroes/heroines who save or try to save lives to stimulate others to achieve an environment where self sacrifice is no longer required, however unlikely that may prove.

Some – many – people do care and yes, of course the Barbara Harrison Prize is a small but long standing tribute to her, for and from some of those.

Appendix 1

The Citation for Jane Harrison's George Cross

The London Gazette: 8 August , 1969

On 8 April 1968, soon after take-off from Heathrow Airport, No. 2 engine of B.O.A.C. Boeing 707 G-ARWE caught fire and subsequently fell from the aircraft, leaving a fierce fire burning at No. 2 engine position. About two and a half minutes later the aircraft made an emergency landing at the airport and the fire on the port wing intensified. Miss Harrison was one of the stewardesses in this aircraft and the duties assigned to her in an emergency were to help the steward at the aft station to open the appropriate rear door and inflate the escape chute and then to assist passengers at the rear of the aircraft to leave in an orderly manner. When the aircraft landed Miss Harrison and the steward concerned opened the rear galley door and inflated the chute, which unfortunately became twisted on the way down so that the steward had to climb down it to straighten it before it could be used. Once out of the aircraft he was unable to return; hence Miss Harrison was left alone to the task of shepherding passengers to the rear door and helping them out of the aircraft. She encouraged some passengers to jump from the machine and pushed others. **With flames and explosions all around her and escape from the tail of the machine impossible she remained at her post. She was finally overcome while trying to save an elderly cripple who was seated in one of the last rows and whose body was found** close to that of the stewardess. Miss Harrison was a very brave young lady who gave her life in utter devotion to duty.

Appendix 2

Dedication of a plaque in memory of BARBARA JANE HARRISON GC 23 October 1970 at 11.30 a.m. at the Chapel of Saint George Heathrow Airport

To commemorate the memory of BOAC Stewardess

BARBARA JANE HARRISON

aged 22 years

who was posthumously awarded the George Cross for courage and selfless devotion to duty in the evacuation of passengers from a blazing Boeing 707 aircraft G-ARWE at Heathrow Airport on 8th April 1968

Passengers praised Miss Harrison's calmness and courage throughout the evacuation. At the last although she could have saved herself, she gave her life attempting to help a crippled passenger to leave the aircraft

In the name of the Father and of the Son and of the Holy Spirit, we dedicate this plaque in thankful memory of Barbara Jane Harrison, to be a lasting memorial of she who faced the final challenge of humanity and was not found wanting.

Appendix 3

Letter announcing
Neville Davis-Gordon's Award

HONOURS – IN CONFIDENCE

10 Downing Street
Whitehall

August 5, 1969

Sir,

  I have the honour to inform you that The Queen
has been graciously pleased to approve the Prime
Minister's recommendation that you be awarded the
British Empire Medal for Gallantry (Civil Division)
(B.E.M.). Your name will therefore appear in a
list of awards to be published in the London Gazette
on the evening of Friday, August 8.

  You will understand that this letter must be
treated as strictly confidential until the evening
of Friday, August 8.

     I am, Sir,

      Your obedient Servant,

       Michael Halls

N. C. Davis-Gordon, Esq.

Appendix 4

The Fate of Whisky Echo

It is hard to imagine, when looking at the photos of the burnt out shell of Whisky Echo, that anything could be salvaged from the wreck.

When the twisted metal was removed from its resting place on runway 05R and was taken behind the BOAC hangars at the airline's engineering base at Hatton Cross, it was difficult to lift the main structure which was so badly damaged that parts just fell off. There was, however, one section which remained intact. This was the nose section of the aircraft including the cockpit.

On 29 August 1969 a Boeing 707-331B, registration number N776TW, belonging to American airline TWA, took off from Rome bound for Athens on flight TW 840. Unknown to the crew two of the passengers on board were members of the Popular Front for the Liberation of Palestine. They hijacked the aircraft and forced the pilot to fly to the Syrian capital, Damascus. Once on the ground the passengers and crew were able to escape via the emergency chutes but two explosive devices were thrown by the hijackers into the cockpit, destroying it but leaving the rest of the aircraft intact. It was found that the main structure was sound enough for the aircraft to be repaired and so a new nose section was sought and found. The last surviving part of Whisky Echo was used to repair N776TW.[1]

The aircraft had its test flight with the new cockpit on 4 December 1969 and flew with the airline for just over ten more years under its new registration, N28714. It was withdrawn from service in March 1980 and stored in Kansas City, Missouri before being sold, three years later, to Boeing. It was moved to

Davis-Monthan Air Force Base in Arizona and was used by the USAF as spares for its KC135E tanker aircraft. The aircraft's registration was only cancelled in March 1984 and so Whisky Echo's nose and cockpit lived on for many years after the rest of its structure had been destroyed.

Notes

Introduction
1. *1968: The Year that Rocked the World* by Mark Kurlansky published by Jonathan Cape, 2004.

Chapter 3
1. Author's conversation with Michael Moore.
2. Author's conversation with Andrew McCarthy.
3. *Time Flies – Heathrow at 60*, Alan Gallop, Sutton Publishing, 2005.

Chapter 4
1. *Enough Rope with Andrew Denton*, ABC TV show in Australia on 5 September 2005.
2. *Daily Telegraph*, Tuesday 9 April 1968.
3. *Daily Express*, Tuesday 9 April 1968
4. Letter from Dorothy Morcom Taylor to Alan Harrison, 3 June 1970.

Chapter 5
1. Information from documents in the National Archives.
2. A sari is one single piece of fabric, six yards long, pleated with the fingers as it is wound around the body, and fixed in place by tucking the top edge into the band of a tight fitting underskirt.
3. Information from documents in the National Archives.
4. ibid.
5. Author's conversations with Andrew McCarthy and Rosalind Chatterley née Unwin.

6. Information from documents in the National Archives.
7. ibid.
8. Author's conversation with Andrew McCarthy.

Chapter 6
1. The Radiochemical Centre, Amersham, later Amersham International.
2. Pacific Standard Time – GMT-8 hours.

Chapter 7
1. Reported in *Daily Mirror* Tuesday 9 April 1968.
2. *Northern Despatch*, 9 April 1968.
3. *The Guardian* front page, 10 April 1968.
4. *The Northern Echo* 10 April 1968.
5. *Northern Despatch*, 11 April 1968.
6. Author's conversation with Kay Haw née Golightly.

Chapter 8
1. The first officer reading out the item and the appropriate crew member confirming that the action had been taken.
2. On this occasion it should have been John Hutchinson.
3. Acting First Officer Hutchinson.
4. The figure was actually 126.
5. Times were shown in GMT rather than British Summer Time which was in force on 8 April.

Chapter 9
1. He was Minister of Transport and Civil Aviation from 1954-55.
2. A hostel for immigrants, which gave accommodation to new arrivals for a maximum of six weeks.
3. Unattributed document in the British Airways museum.
4. An extremely modest man, John had to be persuaded by his wife Jaqi to talk about his award and to allow the photo of him, with his MBE, to be published in this book.

Chapter 10
1. Correspondence from Alan Bishop, Managing Director of EBM Insurance Brokers, West Perth dated 24 September 2007.
2. Author's conversation with Richard Hamond.

3. Author's conversation with Rosalind Chatterley née Unwin.
4. Information from documents found in the National Archives.
5. Author's conversation with Andrew McCarthy.

Chapter 11
1. Worth approximately £10,000 in 2008. Source: Currency converter on the website of the National Archives.
2. Worth approximately £136 in 2008. Source: Currency converter on the website of the National Archives.
3. See www.sghsoldgirls.org.uk

Appendix 4
1. *Boeing 707, 727 and KC-135* by Tony Pither, published by Air Britain Historians Ltd.

Bibliography

Books

Bish, Pete and Piket, Brian, *Heathrow ATC – the First 50 Years*, Zebedee Balloon Service Ltd, 2005

Crocker, David, *Dictionary of Aeronautical English*, Peter Collin Publishing, 1999

Gallop, Alan, *Time Flies – Heathrow at 60*, Sutton Publishing, 2005

Gunston, Bill, *Early Jetliners*, Phoebus Publishing, 1980

Job, Macarthur, *Air Disaster Volume 1*, Aerospace Publications Pty Ltd, 1994

Lloyd, Alwyn T., *Boeing 707 & AWACS*, Arms & Armour Press, 1987

Penrose, Harald, *Wings Across the World – An Illustrated History of British Airways*, Cassell Ltd, 1980

Pither, Tony, *Boeing 707, 727 and KC-135*, Air Britain Historians Ltd, 1999

Road, Alan, *The Facts about an Airline, featuring British Airways*, G. Whizzard Publications, 1978

Rolls-Royce, *The Jet Engine*, Rolls-Royce Ltd, 1973

Sherwood, Philip, *The History of Heathrow*, Hillingdon Libraries, 1990

Winchester, Jim, *Airlife's Classic Airliners – Boeing 707/720*, Airlife Publishing Ltd, 2002

Woodley, Charles, *BOAC – An Illustrated History*, Tempus Publishing, 2004

Other Sources

Magazines
BOAC News
Horizon
Paris Match
This England

Newspapers
Coventry Evening Telegraph
Daily Express
Daily Mail
Daily Mirror
Daily Sketch
Evening Standard
Northern Despatch
The Birmingham Post
The Daily Telegraph
The Evening News
The Guardian
The Herald (Melbourne)
The Northern Echo
The Staines and Egham News
The West Australian
Yorkshire Post

Index